What people are saying about

Bodies Arising

Nicole Schnackenberg skilfully and compassionately presents a pathway to healing and hope for sincere practitioners ready to move into a more expanded understanding of who they are and what it means to live in a body. This book is an excellent addition to the growing body of work aimed at dismantling the damaging imperatives of culture and the painful consequences of spiritual hunger.
Christina Sell, author of *Yoga from the Inside Out: Making Peace with Your Body Through Yoga* and *My Body is a Temple: Yoga as a Path of Wholeness*

Nicole Schnackenberg's beautiful book *Bodies Arising* will help many people rediscover their true self and heal their struggles with body acceptance and self-love.
Dr Ramdesh Kaur, author of *The Body Temple: Kundalini Yoga for Body Acceptance, Eating Disorders & Radical Self-Love*

T0163006

Bodies Arising

Fall in Love with your Body and Remember your Divine Essence

Bodies Arising

Fall in Love with your Body and Remember your Divine Essence

Nicole Schnackenberg

BOOKS

Winchester, UK
Washington, USA

JOHN HUNT PUBLISHING

First published by O-Books, 2019
O-Books is an imprint of John Hunt Publishing Ltd., 3 East St., Alresford,
Hampshire SO24 9EE, UK
office@jhpbooks.com
www.johnhuntpublishing.com
www.o-books.com

For distributor details and how to order please visit the 'Ordering' section on our website.

ISBN: 978 1 78904 260 3
978 1 78904 261 0 (ebook)
Library of Congress Control Number: 2019930798

A CIP catalogue record for this book is available from the British Library.

Design: Stuart Davies

UK: Printed and bound by CPI Group (UK) Ltd, Croydon, CR0 4YY
US: Printed and bound by Thomson-Shore, 7300 West Joy Road, Dexter, MI 48130

We operate a distinctive and ethical publishing philosophy in
all areas of our business, from our global network of authors to
production and worldwide distribution.

Contents

The fact is that there is nothing more beautiful, more worthy or more conscious than you.
Yogi Bhajan

For Ruth

Foreword by Theresa Cheung

Physical appearance has never been so centre-stage in our lives as it is today. We live in a selfie-based culture where the compulsion to look movie star ready on our newsfeeds, videos and profiles is pervasive. It seems as if the camera and photo lens is constantly on. Research has clearly shown that the feelings of ugliness and self-loathing that come with aspiring to this impossible bodily ideal is responsible for an ever-growing epidemic of depression, eating disorders and body image problems.

Something urgently needs to be done to help us reconnect with our bodies. It would not be an understatement to say that discontent with the way we look can destroy happiness and devastate lives. There are many books and courses which address body hatred and how to heal it through diet and psychological approaches. However, as therapeutic as these treatments are, they are not sustainable because they look at the symptoms and not the cause. The only sure-fire way to address body image problems is by looking at the root cause which is a hunger and thirst for self-love and a deeper meaning to our lives.

In *Bodies Arising*, Nicole Schnackenberg has written an important book that should be required reading for everyone today, especially for young people. It turns the spotlight on a spiritual understanding of our bodies and body hatred. Nicole explains that to not love your body is to not love yourself, and that this destructive lack of self-love can be cured through finding a deeper sense of meaning and purpose in your life. The way to find that sense of deep meaning and purpose is through reconnecting to yourself as a spiritual being and recognising your body as a beautiful physical representation of who you truly are: Your spiritual essence.

The emphasis in this book on the body as a means to reconnect with our spiritual nature is what makes it truly unique. All too often in mystical, religious or New Age teaching the emphasis is on the power of the mind or our thoughts to discover our true spiritual meaning. Bodily needs are either dismissed or regarded as base or carnal with the sins of the flesh being a familiar refrain. Material concerns are regarded as a distraction from our true spiritual essence. The body is not valued or loved and is considered a poor companion for the mind. Even the New Age mind-body revolution, where thoughts are believed to impact our bodily health, assigns a subordinate role to the body with the body blindly following the directive of our thoughts. *Bodies Arising* brilliantly corrects that misconception and puts the body centre-stage in personal transformation. It shows that our bodies are just as important, perhaps even more so, than our thoughts. We need to listen to our bodies, appreciate and love them 'warts and all', because our bodies are as much our spiritual teachers as our thoughts and our feelings are.

Perhaps the selfie culture we live in has arisen for a reason. The body denied spiritual expression for too long is trying to get us to notice it in any way it can. This book is written by someone who has truly listened to their body and wants everyone to discover their own body-loving, self-healing light as she has. As someone who has survived a serious eating disorder, Nicole is the perfect guide for the life-changing journey this book takes you on. Whether you are suffering from an eating disorder or not you will learn how to fall in love with your body as an authentic expression of who you truly are. Along the way, Nicole shares her inspiring story of recovery and shows that although body image problems can feel like the end of our lives they may, in fact, be a new beginning and a rebirth. They are a spiritual awakening, the darkness before the dawn, a desperate cry for attention from our bodies urging us to discover meaning from the inside out and the outside in.

Theresa Cheung, Sunday Times *bestselling author of* 21 Rituals to Change Your Life *(Watkins) and* Answers from Heaven *(Piatkus)*
www.theresacheung.com

Chapter One

Remember That the Body is Not You

To identify the self with a body is learned. It is not innate.

We come into this world without a sense of being or having a body. The body of a baby is not a body *for* the baby. It is simply what 'is', and even to say this is a bit too much.

For the baby, in fact, there *is* no body. And no nursery, no blanket. Nothing. No 'thing' at all.

There is no experience of being a person for the baby. There is no notion of a being one person 'over here' in a relationship with other people 'out there'.

Rather, the experience of a baby is one of seamless aliveness. Sensations coming and going, perceptions emerging and dissolving.

The breath comes in and out through the baby's mouth and nostrils. Yet, there is neither mouth nor nostrils for the baby, neither air nor breath. The chest rises and falls as the baby breathes. Yet, there is no chest for the baby, and no distinction between the rise and the fall of it.

What is innate are sensations. From the moment an infant is born, they experience sensations and the ability to respond to these sensations. Some of these sensations are displayed through their expressive behaviour. The infant experiences hunger and begins to cry. They experience satiety and the crying ends.

The baby has no experience of edges. It is not until a baby is around four to five months old—and sometimes, it is later than this—that they begin to have any kind of a notion that they are a separate self at all. It then takes another ten months or so for the baby to begin to recognise themselves in the mirror.

There is a difference between feeling a connection with the sensations of the body and a belief that the self *is* the body. To have a lived experience of the body is totally natural. To believe that the body *is* the self can lead to tremendous suffering and pain.

For some people, the belief that the body is the self can lead to battles with and against the appearance of this body. Some people turn to dieting and excessive exercise, others to cosmetic surgery and endless mirror-gazing. Some people turn to suicide. On the surface of it, they appear to take their own lives because they believe that the way they look says everything about who they are.

We digress from having no sense whatsoever that the body has anything to do with the self to believing that the body *is* the self. Sometimes, we make this digression in a very short space of time. Children as young as three years old have been found to lament over their perceived ugliness and to hate themselves because of the way they think they look.

We become aware of how we look as we move out of infancy. We often become particularly aware of our appearance in adolescence—the period of life during which diagnoses such as eating disorders and body dysmorphic disorder (BDD) are the most common.

When the appearance of the body is derided by thoughts, experiences of sensing the body and attaching identity to the body can become very topsy-turvy. Essentially, there is a pinning of the identity on to the physical body. At the same time, there is a reduced ability to sense the body. The lived experience of the body is muted. Attention to the appearance of the physical body is heightened.

We will return to this again and again, to this concept of the lived experience of the body from the inside—our interoceptive awareness. Interoceptive awareness is made up of the impressions in the body of the heartbeat, breathing, hunger, satiety, temperature, tension, pain, blood pressure, blood sugar level, sexual arousal, and many other internal phenomena.

Our ability to interocept—and to respond to the interoceptive signals we experience—is vital to our survival. As infants, we were unable to meet our own basic needs. If we were hungry, we were unable to leave our cot and prepare ourselves a bottle of milk or find our own way to our mother's breast. It was necessary that we first noticed the hunger and then made this hunger known through our expressive behaviour, perhaps through crying. This cry was designed by Mother Nature to obtain the attention of our caregivers, to bring them to us.

This was not a conscious process. For the baby, there is neither hunger nor milk. There is only whatever is happening. There is simply 'hunger' happening and 'crying' happening in once-seamless beingness. Aliveness calls out to aliveness and invites aliveness into itself. The baby's cry invites soothing or rejection or curiosity or a vast number of alternative possibilities.

The kind of response the baby receives is contingent on many factors: How in touch with their own interoceptive signals the caregivers are; the presence of any past trauma; the living situation of the caregivers (e.g., how safe, well-nourished, warm, and/or loved they feel); the support network around them, and so on.

Some of us would have experienced 'good enough' caregiving as infants, to use psychoanalyst and paediatrician Donald Winnicott's term. This does not mean that our caregivers responded to our needs one-hundred per cent perfectly, one-hundred per cent of the time—maybe more like thirty per cent of the time, according to specialists in the field of developmental psychology. Good enough is good enough. Others would have had the experience of their needs being met more or less than this, sometimes much more or much less.

There is a direct relationship between the meeting of our needs as infants and an emergent sense of safety in the body. This sense of safety is a somatic experience. It takes place in the muscles, the viscera, the breathing cycle... potentially in every crevice and corner of the infant's physicality.

A sense of safety in the body as an infant is strongly related to attachment. Attachment describes the way in which human beings connect with and attune to other human beings, initially, in the context of the primary caregiving relationship. Some of us would have had secure attachments with our primary caregivers. We would have had the experience of our needs being met, of being held in mind, and of having a secure base from which to go out and explore the world. Others of us would have had less secure attachments, perhaps experiencing an emotional disconnect between ourselves and those caring for us.

There was an interesting experiment conducted in 1985 by Donovan and Leavitt. They found that when infants who had been classified as securely attached were left by their mothers, they typically began to demonstrate distress through their expressive behaviours, such as through crying. At the same time, their heart rate went up. When the infants who had been classified as insecurely attached were left by their mothers, on the other hand, they tended not to cry or demonstrate visible distress. Their heart rate, importantly, went up in the very same way. The infants classified as insecurely attached had learned to ignore the interoceptive signal of their heartbeat; or at least, they had learned not to express increased heart rate through their behaviour. Perhaps they unconsciously understood that crying did not bring the caregiver to them, or that the caregiver's presence was not entirely safe. Perhaps they learned that their crying would scare Mummy or Daddy away. Maybe they unconsciously learned to cut themselves off from sensations of distress in the body.

Neuroscientist Stephen Porges shed some very interesting light on some of these processes through his polyvagal theory. He hypothesises that we have three lines of defence when it comes to feeling unsafe and being under threat. Of course, these threats do not have to be threats to our physical safety.

Emotional threats are just as powerful and terrifying, such as when we reached out for comfort as infants and did not receive it.

Our three lines of defence are linked to the vagus nerve. The vagus nerve is often referred to as the 'wanderer'. It is the longest cranial nerve and has branches that 'wander' throughout the body. It is part of the parasympathetic nervous system and sends messages both to and away from the brain and spinal cord. Very interestingly, it is linked with the skeletal muscles of the face, middle ear, and larynx, and therefore, plays an important role in facial expressions, talking, swallowing, and hearing. A very intriguing nerve indeed.

When we believe ourselves to be in danger, Porges hypothesises that we first utilise our ventral vagal complex for social engagement. We attempt to engage or appease the other primarily through our facial expressions and voice as infants. If this does not work (if we are unable to engage or appease our caregiver with our smiles, gurgles, and so on) the ventral vagal complex is deactivated and the sympathetic (fight, flight, freeze, or fawn) nervous system is aroused. We attempt to either fight the danger, escape it (flight), become invisible (freeze), or please the other by acting servilely (fawn).

If this line of defence does not work, we move into the third line of defence. It is clear at this moment that the dangerous thing — whatever that might be — is going to happen. We are certain that we cannot change or escape the external environment, nor can we alter how we feel about it. An unconscious, vagal system-based decision is therefore made that it would be better if we were not 'present' to witness whatever is happening or is going to happen. That would be unbearable. Thus, the dorsal vagal system is switched on. At this point, many systems of the body shut down, we dissociate, and we no longer have an experience of the sensations of the body.

A reduced sense of the lived experience of the body — a kind

7

of dissociation from sensation—would appear to be at the heart of many appearance-focused struggles. Research is increasingly showing that people with diagnoses of anorexia, bulimia, and BDD have poorer interoceptive awareness than those without these diagnoses. It is possible that this reduced interoceptive awareness exists within and across many other—if not all—manifestations of appearance-focused battles.

The practices that so many of us engage in when we are trying to alter the physical appearance of our body often ignore and dampen our interoceptive signals even further. You can perhaps imagine how catastrophic this can become if one's interoceptive awareness is already poor. Dieting is a perfect example of this. Each time we deny the body of the food it needs, we ignore interoceptive signals like hunger and blood sugar imbalance. Excessive exercise is another example. Each time we push our bodies far beyond their physical limits, we shove down interoceptive signals, such as fatigue and pain.

These interoceptive signals do not exist only to let us know when we are hungry, cold, tired, and so on. Interoceptive signals are the very language of our emotional lives.

We become disconnected from our emotions to the extent that we are cut off from our interoceptive signals. As neuroscientist Antonio Damasio describes it, *'Emotions use the body as their theatre.'* We only know how we are feeling emotionally because of how we are feeling physically. The next time you feel angry, for example, ask yourself how you know. You will find that you know through and in the sensations of the body. Expressive behaviours, such as clenching your teeth or shouting, may follow these sensations. The thought, 'I am feeling angry,' may follow these sensations. But the anger is not the behaviours, nor is it the thoughts. The anger is the sensations themselves.

Emotions are bodily sensations. They are sensual energy in motion. Our emotions are an intrinsic element of our sense of aliveness. Without them, the seeming object that is our body is, experientially, an empty shell.

To have a sense of being cut off from one's emotions is to feel dead inside, to feel disconnected from a sense of self. It is to experience a loss of a sense of connection with others.

We experience emotions from the moment we are born— and surely, before this—yet, we do not have any concepts or language for these emotions in infancy. They are implicit, procedural experiences stored in the primitive and limbic parts of the brain. Our emotions are intrinsically tied to our interoceptive awareness, our lived experience of the body. From the very first few moments of life, our interoceptive signals are also intrinsically bound to our relationships. As tiny infants, this was a seamless experience, as we did not have any sense of our body being separate from our caregiver. The breast that brought the milk to our lips when we cried with hunger was as much 'us' as the lips themselves. Then, at a certain point, we began to have the experience of our lips over 'here' and our mother's breast over 'there'. Our mother became a separate object, a separate person.

This is assuming that all goes well. Infants are only able to individuate successfully and develop a robust, separate sense of self in the context of secure attachment relationships. As we will explore in much more depth as we move through this book, infants who do not pass through this developmental stage of individuation can have the ongoing, unconscious experience that their body is synonymous with the body of their caregiver. They may remain enmeshed. They may have no sense, psychically or emotionally, of where they begin-and-end and where their caregiver begins and ends. Importantly, human beings need to find out where they begin-and-end and other objects begin-and-end in order to engage in relationship with them.

It is possible that this is one of the reasons why diagnoses like anorexia most commonly emerge in adolescence and are more common in the female population (although males are increasingly struggling with this and other appearance-focused struggles). At this stage of development, the female body can feel as though it is coming to more closely resemble that of the mother's; breasts mature, menstruation begins, and so on. By starving the breasts and the menstruation away, the girl halts becoming a woman and assumes a largely androgynous body which is neither strongly male nor strongly female; thus, unconsciously asserting separation from the body of her mother.

At a certain point in infancy, there is a developing sense of being inside, and possessing, a body. There also emerges a developing connectedness to that body. This is facilitated by the repeated experience of bodily care provided by the caregiver. As we are held, fed, washed, tucked into our cots, cuddled, and so on, we begin to develop a sense of our edges. We begin to separate the arms which embrace us from the body which is being embraced. We seem to become a 'something' in a cot in relation to another 'something' (the caregiver) out there in the world. In this way, our sensations and perceptions become embedded—or, rather, embodied—in flesh and blood.

It takes an infant around four to five months to reach this stage of development. Before this, the infant oscillates between the experience of being one-with-all-things and the experience of being a separate self. Eventually, these oscillations lessen, and the infant comes to an experience of being *a person in a body* having a relationship with others in other bodies. The infant arrives at an experience of having an inside, an outside, and a body schema (an internal representation of their body parts in space). This sense of having and being a body does not happen autonomously. It is enabled by, and occurs within, the embodied presence of a caregiver or caregivers.

Over time, the infant finds different ways of adapting to the environment to survive physiologically, psychologically, and emotionally. One such survival mechanism is the development of a false self. Winnicott wrote extensively about the development of the false self within the infant-primary caregiver relationship. This self is given the opportunity to develop from the very first hours of life.

In the early stages of its development, the infant primarily acts on spontaneous impulses, with the source of such spontaneity being their true Self. Interoceptive signals and emotions are experienced and expressed freely and with abandon. The primary caregiver then meets these spontaneous impulses in either a 'good enough' or 'not good enough' way, to use Winnicott's terms. The 'good enough' response meets the spontaneity of the infant repeatedly; thus, providing a space for their true Self to flourish. The 'not good enough' response fails to accommodate the infant's spontaneity. Instead, the primary caregiver repeatedly substitutes the infant's spontaneous gestures and emotions with their own. Most usually, the infant complies and there is an emergence of a false self that is more readily able to meet the needs and desires of the caregiver.

If the infant is continually unable to act spontaneously from their true Self, they may quickly learn that their true Self is not acceptable and is, therefore, to be hidden away. The true desires, needs, and personality of the infant may, therefore, be relinquished to the shadows.

Infants learn how to read the faces and mimic the gestures of their caregivers within the first forty-two minutes of life. Infants are geniuses at adapting their facial expressions, body language, and behaviour to keep their caregivers close to them. Infants and young children will adapt who they truly are to a high magnitude to remain connected to their caregivers. They will become a false self, if they need to. This will happen unconsciously. In the process, it may seem as though the person loses touch with who they are.

We can think of our true Self as our spontaneous sense of aliveness. Or, we might like to call it Pure Awareness, Consciousness, Beingness... Love.

In many ways, appearance-focused struggles could be said to be direct manifestations of the false self. The spontaneity and innate sense of aliveness are denied. The interoceptive signals and emotions are suppressed. The energy fixates on the creation of a self that more readily meets the lovability standards of the primary caregiver or other key figures in the person's life.

The way our true Self or false self emerges will depend on a wide host of complex factors embedded in our culture, such as conditioning, physiology, sensitivities, beliefs, and all manner of other things. To lay all the blame for appearance-focused struggles at the feet of early attachment relationships—or, indeed, in the lap of any theory, relationship, or circumstance—would be oversimplifying the whole matter. This is not to deny, however, that the body-mind is deeply shaped by its environment not only from the very moment the infant is born, but also—as research is increasingly indicating—within the womb.

At some point in their development, the infant comes to recognise themselves in the mirror. This recognition most usually happens after the false self has already started to emerge. It was Jacques Lacan's view that the infant is born with a fragmented body. At what he calls the 'Mirror Stage', the infant beholds an image of wholeness in the body—they see a seamless entity, which they ascribe with the lived-sense of 'I'.

The image of wholeness experienced in the mirror counteracts the infant's experience of the fragmented body. The infant, thus, assumes an identity which is implicitly linked with the body they view in the mirror. The infant 'becomes' a complete, coherent object within the cacophony of seeming 'other' objects in the world.

From here, the infant begins to further separate their experience into categories, such as plants, animals, foods, toys, humans, and so on. That which is pre-Mirror Stage is pre-symbolic. It simply is what it is. It is a seamless experience of sensations and perceptions. Whatever is happening is happening. There is no you. There is no me. No objectified world, in fact. Suddenly, the infant is thrust into a seeming reality, in which everything belongs in a category and is a symbol of meaning; a world in which reality which is not symbolised (made conscious) through language is not deemed, in the societal dominant discourse, to be real.

During the stage of the identification of the mirror image as the 'I', we find ourselves to be an aesthetic object among other aesthetic objects. There appears to be a profound bereavement at this stage. *I look into the mirror and see myself—or so, I believe. I look around me and I see the Other in a myriad of forms and guises. How do I reach from inside 'here' to outside 'there'? How do I connect and relate? How do I become/remain a part of your world and how do you become/remain a part of mine? What am I looking at when I look at you? And what do you see when you are looking at me?*

The dichotomy is that this process of individuation is a crucial stage of human development. To understand that our body is not the body of our primary caregiver, and to come to an embodied sense of our own edges, is vital for an experience of autonomy and agency. Fundamentally, it also makes the lived experience of person-to-person relationship possible. Alongside this sits the truth that the true Self is *not the body*. Your essential essence is not the body that ages and dies. Your essential nature is spirit, not flesh. Your essential nature is Love.

At the core of all the major religions and spiritual traditions is the same mystical knowledge and metaphysical truth—an experience and lived understanding of the existence of a Self beyond the body-mind. In its essence, the perennial philosophy brings us back to the questions mystics and saints have asked themselves throughout the ages: *What is it that dies? Is our essential nature subject to birth and death?* In many ways the infant is a mystic—experiencing themselves as being one with all phenomena without any sense of impermanence. The infant then moves into a necessary sense of separation before returning, at some point, to the knowledge of their impermanence. This may happen before or after death. A great many human beings, in fact, seem to go through a whole physical lifetime without ever remembering (or perhaps even questioning) who they truly are.

Many of us have assumed that our identity is the body and the mind without ever having questioned this. The idea that the 'I' we take ourselves to be is a bundle of thoughts and a mass of bones/blood/viscera etc. is only that—only an idea; only, itself, a thought.

Somehow, we seem to retain (at least in part) a sense of the Self beyond the thoughts we think and the body we feel. There appears to be a residual sense—sometimes, buried under layers of conditioning—that we *are not the body that ages and dies*. At the same time, there is the feeling of a void in which this sense of connection has been 'lost' or forgotten. We try to get back to this sense of connection, and to fill this void, in all manner of ways—through relationships, possessions, careers, substances, food, the denial of food, the alteration of the physical body and many other ways besides.

This book is largely about the journey back to our true Selves. Unlike in infancy when this experience was unconscious, however, the journey back renders it consciously known. This true Self could equally be called Aliveness, Beingness, Freedom, Peace, Oneness, and Love. To be more accurate, it is a book about a sort of non-journey—a book about finding that we already are that which we seek. Peace and Love are not things we must find or return to. Peace and Love are who we are.

A Note on Perfectionism

Fundamentally, we are both perfect and imperfect. The truth lies at the centre of the dichotomy. The true Self is the awareness which permeates all seeming things. It is both darkness and light, suffering and joy. The word *Guru* encapsulates this beautifully. It is comprised of the word *Gu* meaning *cave* or *darkness*, and *ru*, meaning *light*. The *Guru*, therefore, is the *light in the darkness*. Jung explained it in a similar way with his analogy of the black sun. The darkness *is* the light. Our seeming imperfections are themselves the light; our perfection lies within them. Embrace and welcome with open arms all that you think is imperfect about yourself and you will discover exactly what I mean. The following little exercise might support you in this endeavour.

Embracing 'Imperfection' Meditation

Find a quiet, comfortable place where you know you will not be disturbed. If it helps, call your allies to mind—those people (or animals) who have touched your life (whether you have met them or not, whether they are alive or dead). Surround yourself with the sense of their loving, compassionate support.

Call to mind a part of yourself you would label 'imperfect', a part of yourself you have been trying to make perfect in some way. It might be an appearance-based 'imperfection' or something about your personality, behaviour, or character. Stay with the aspect you have identified and begin to sense where the lived experience of this aspect resides in the body. Feel deeply into the associated sensation or sensations in the body, noticing any resistance and welcoming this with open arms also. Welcome these sensations as though they were frightened children, desperate for your attention and your loving, non-judgemental, compassionate embrace.

Thank your perceived imperfection for being there. Thank it out loud if you would like to: 'Thank you, fat on my thighs, for being there.' Notice the sensations this ignites in your body. Stay with these sensations. Place the full light of your attention on these sensations, as though they were the most interesting and important phenomena in all the world.

Notice any resistance in your body as you thank your perceived imperfection. Feel into and embrace the sensation of this resistance. Repeat your extension of thanks to your perceived imperfection—again, out loud if you feel able: 'Thank you, fat on my thighs, for being there.'

Again, feel into any sensations, particularly sensations of resistance. Repeat this process until you can no longer find any resistance in your body. If you have been engaged in this practice for a long while and are continuing to feel waves of resistance, thank your resistance for trying to keep you safe but explain that you no longer need it: 'Thank you for being here, resistance. I know you are trying to keep me safe from feeling the fat on my thighs. I know you are trying to keep me safe from this because you understand that my fear of fat on my thighs is rooted in my fear of being unlovable.' Feel deeply into any sensation-based responses and repeat if you feel able. Otherwise, thank both your fear and your resistance, and assure both that you will be back another time in the not-too-distant future to spend time with them. And make sure you keep your word!

Chapter Two

Walk Towards Fear

As body-minds, we are wired for survival. If our caregivers do not respond to our expressive behaviours when we are infants, we will die. Yet, the dance of attunement would appear to encompass much more than this attempt to keep the body-mind organism alive.

In the 1950s and 1960s, a researcher named Harry Harlow lamented the fact that very little scientific research had been dedicated to the subject of love. In his most well-known experiment, Harlow gave young rhesus monkeys the choice of various wire-mesh 'mothers'. One of these wire-mesh mothers had a feeding bottle attached, while another mother was wrapped in soft terrycloth. If the monkeys were only interested in receiving food, it would have followed that they would have spent much—if, perhaps, not all—of their time with the wire-mesh, attached-bottle mothers. This was not the case. The monkeys overwhelmingly preferred to spend time with their terrycloth mothers, visiting the wire-mesh mothers only to feed. Harlow's work beautifully complements that of John Bowlby, who believed that bonding (in this case, in humans) occurs not only because of met physiological needs (such as hunger) but also due to a need for intimate contact. Harlow, Bowlby, and many others before and since have postulated that human beings are intrinsically wired not only for survival, but also for love.

The brain of the infant does not know the difference between food and the mother. 'Food' and 'mother' are absorbed as one seamless experience. Neither is the infant's brain able to make a distinction between the contact-comfort and love it receives, and the mother who provides it. In this way, food is synonymous with the mother, and both are synonymous with love and survival. For the infant:

Food = Survival
Food = Mother
Mother = Survival
Love = Survival

As we began to explore in Chapter One, we are not born with a sense of separation from other people and objects. Our experience in early infancy, rather, is that of a wash of sensations and perceptions arising and dissolving. Gradually, we come to have a sense that there is an identity 'in here' and a world 'out there'. We come to believe that we 'have' and even 'are' a body.

Before we have a sense of being a separate self, we have a sense of being intimately connected with everything around us. We are the breath, the feeding bottle, the wind, the blanket—all of it. There is no separation between any of it. And a lack of separation is, perhaps, the best description of love.

When we explore our experience, we find that, at the root of all our fears, is the root fear of being unloved. The notion of being unloved is synonymous with death. Every fibre of our being knows this. Human beings can and do die of a lack of love, whatever age they may be.

Any experience within which we are treated as though we are not lovable, therefore, is utterly terrifying to the infant. This template of unlovability being synonymous with the terror of death is a foundational template of the human experience. Thus, when we experience the sense that we are anything less than lovable, every fibre of our being reacts in enormous terror, in an experience of *'nameless dread'*, to use psychoanalyst Wilfred Bion's phrase. We react adaptively both by trying to save ourselves and trying to soothe ourselves. We try to save ourselves by attempting to become lovable and by stamping the perceived unlovable aspects out. And we try to soothe ourselves in all manner of ways. The use of substances, overeating and under-eating, and engaging in compulsive, repetitive behaviours are just a few examples.

Our fear of not being loved does not belong to or spring from the true Self. The true Self *is* Love and fears nothing. This fear is the fear of the body-mind organism. This fear might show up in a million different ways. Yet, when we trace it back to its origin, we arrive at the absolute terror that we, as a body-mind, might be unlovable. The sense that we are unlovable places us, in our direct lived experience, on the cusp of emotional, psychological and physical death.

There is a pervasive societal myth that we can become more lovable by changing the appearance of the physical body. This myth feeds neatly into the core, foundational terror of being unlovable, and therefore, being perpetually on the edge of annihilation. If we have any sense that we might not be completely lovable exactly as we are, we will look for ways to become more lovable to remain connected to our caregivers, to *be safe and to survive.* If we look to society, we are likely to come across (although, we do not need to 'come across' it—most of us are saturated in it) the message that we can become more lovable by becoming thinner, more muscular, or whatever appearance project it might be. We then become tangled up in the fear of gaining weight/not losing weight etc. Yet, the root fear is the fear of being unloved.

I invite you to try it. Take any fear linked to the appearance of your body or otherwise and keep tracing it back until you are unable to go any further. If you continue to follow the fear to its root, you will find that it is absolutely embedded in the evolutionary fear of physical non-survival and/or the terror of being unlovable and unloved.

My fear of being ugly, for example, consumed me for many years of my early life. I tried to run away from the seemingly unbearable prospect that I might be ugly. I ploughed all my energy into changing my physical appearance to undo that ugliness. I wasn't even striving for beauty. I just didn't want to continue to be the monster I believed myself to be. I yearned for the possibility, at least, that I might be worthy of love.

In early adolescence, I received a diagnosis of anorexia and, later, of body dysmorphic disorder. The plan of action in terms of my treatment was for me to ignore the sense of my ugliness, to distract myself from it, and to fight against it. I replaced the fear of being ugly with the fear of the *feeling* of ugliness. Still, I was locked in fear. Still, I was fighting and running. Still, I felt like a monster inside.

At a certain point, after many years of fighting first my ugliness and then my *feeling* of being ugly, it was clear to me that I was getting nowhere. Some of the external behaviours, such as spending hours in front of the mirror, had dropped away. Yet, I continued to feel monstrous, unworthy, despicable, and unlovable.

At a certain point, I felt a strong invitation from life to stop running, to turn around and to run *towards* my ugliness. It was the only option left, the only action I hadn't attempted. I had tried to 'fix' my appearance. I had tried covering up all the mirrors in the house. I had tried to ban myself from looking up dermatological treatments on the Internet and many, many other things besides. But I hadn't tried putting down my sword and walking headlong into my sense of ugliness, totally unarmed.

I ceased trying to fix my ugliness and began to move towards it. As I came closer, my ugliness seemed to become bigger and even more terrifying. I thought I would explode into a thousand tiny pieces with the pain of it. The agony of the sense of my ugliness seemed to be burning me alive. The sensations of panic came in massive waves, crashing through my whole body as I actively entertained the possibility that I may indeed be hideously ugly (and, therefore, to my mind, utterly unlovable) and always would be.

I was not staying with the sense of my ugliness to escape from it. That would have been more avoidance. I had tried in the past to 'welcome' my ugliness in the desperate hope that this might make it go away. This had been just another layer of avoidance; albeit, a subtler one.

The invitation was to drop any semblance of an agenda. It was an invitation for a complete willingness to welcome any possibility, whatever that might look like. If it meant I discovered that I was the most ugly and monstrous thing to have ever walked this Earth, so be it. If it meant I went mad with the pain of it, so be it. It had to be a total welcoming of my feeling of ugliness, exactly as it was, without any wish to change it. Not ever. I had to be willing to stay with this sense of my ugliness, hold it in my arms, and actively embrace it for the rest of my life, if this were to be the way of things. That was the deal I felt I was being offered. And somehow, after all the years of perpetual avoidance, it was a deal I was willing to take.

So, I moved closer and closer to ugliness. I allowed all the sensations and perceptions in relation to this ugliness to rise without distracting myself from them or trying to stuff them down. I allowed any resistance to be there, too, and I felt into this, also. I uttered a 'yes' to each sensation and perception as it arose, without discrimination or reserve.

The sense that I was ugly filled every cell of my body. It saturated every corner and crevice of my personhood. I sat there in my bedroom and I let it consume everything I felt myself to be.

I quivered and gave up my false self—my identity—for dead. No flowers. No procession. No funeral. Just me alone in my bedroom, dying to myself.

As I truly accepted that I was hideous and ugly and always would be, the waves of terror seemed to fizzle away somewhere. I waited with bated breath for the next wave. It did not come.

I sat there in my bedroom and felt a total absence of the

terror I had been carrying around pretty much my whole life. I continued to welcome the ugliness but could no longer find the feeling of it. I searched the sensations of my body and found only stillness. I looked into my thoughts and found only the absence of thought. I looked into the mirror and welcomed the experience of ugliness I expected to inevitably arise. It did not come.

In that moment, I knew with absolute clarity and complete certainty that I was not ugly, and I never had been. It was not a realisation of thought or body. It was a falling back into something that I, as Awareness, had always been and always known.

I do not know how long I sat there, since this was an experience outside of the usual seeming restraints of time and space. I experienced myself as all things and as nothing. It was as though I had expanded to contain everything in the room and, at the same time, was the room itself and everything beyond the room. It suddenly seemed to be a somewhat comical idea that I would even *identify* with a body, let alone agonise because it was perceived to be ugly. This comedy was not formed by thought. The whole experience was outside of thought. The body began to laugh and cry simultaneously.

It is no exaggeration to say that life was never the same after this experience, nor do I think it ever could be. In that moment of truly welcoming ugliness with open arms, it completely dissolved. Each time it has re-emerged since, I have taken this as a clear and beautiful reminder that I am avoiding and resisting emotions, events and experiences in my life. These are always linked to my root fear of being unlovable, which is begging to be seen and to have its story told. It has been my experience that any fear I embrace with the same unconditional acceptance I afforded ugliness that day in my bedroom does not stick around, certainly in its present form, for very long at all. Rather it transmutes into light. It assimilates into my sense of wholeness.

Of course, the root of my fear of being ugly was my fear of being unlovable. It was the fear of complete emotional and psychological annihilation. In the very same moment in which I knew, with absolute certainty, that I was not ugly, I had the unmistakable knowledge that I was totally lovable, exactly as I was. Not because I was a good body-mind but because I was Love itself, and so were all the people from whom I had longed for love.

We instinctively know that a lack of separation is love. This is one reason why every iota of our being attaches to our primary caregivers when we are infants, and why we say that we 'fall in love' and describe an experience of becoming one with another, of dissolving into them, and of them dissolving into us, somehow.

Yet, for so many body-minds in our current society, this truth has been temporarily veiled behind a mythical separate self. A large part of this separate self is perceived to be the physical body. And a large aspect of the perception of the physical body is tangled up with its appearance. Layer on to this a further myth that the body must look a certain way if we are to be loved, and we have a recipe for intense suffering of the body-mind. In some people, this may manifest as dieting, spending a long time in front of the mirror or at the gym, buying certain clothes, or other such things. For others, it may lead to a search for cosmetic surgery, dentistry, or dermatology. Some may be diagnosed with a mental health condition like anorexia, bulimia, or BDD.

Seeking to change the physical appearance of the body is no different than any other form of seeking. Seeking is the attempt of the separate self to collapse back into Love because it believes it is outside of this Love somehow. The separate self harbours the notion that it wants all manner of things—to gain more muscle, to clear up the skin, to lose weight, to have smaller ears—but all it is ever seeking is the *end* of seeking, an experience of the Love it intrinsically is.

The body-mind has been repeatedly told (both explicitly and implicitly) since birth by parents, family members, teachers, and peers that life revolves around separation. First, there is the body. We are conditioned to believe that our essential nature is located inside the body; that it hears through the ears, for example, and sees through the eyes. We are taught that our essential nature thinks through the mind. Our existence gradually comes to have a whole story attached to it. A name, a remembered past, a supposed future, a personality, likes and dislikes, the ability to accept and reject objects and circumstances... so many things.

Society at large is permeated with the sense that we must protect the false self we take ourselves to be. The world is cruel, and you need to be tough to make it through. You'd better get the best grades, smile, have a talent and excel at it, have an interesting personality, and live a life that others can judge worth living. Much of society also expounds the notion that all of the possibilities you can be and have are totally within your control. A particularly pervasive myth is that the appearance of your body is within your control and that you need to have a 'beautiful' body to be worthy of love.

Return now to your direct experience. Forget what you have been told. Simply stay with your experience in this present moment. Close your eyes if it helps you focus. Have a sense of sinking deep into your heart centre on each long exhalation. Place your awareness on the present moment—on whatever your experience is *right now*. In truth, it is a *collapse* of focus, a total openness to whatever is rising and falling right now. Your thoughts—including thoughts that suggest a personal entity inside the body-mind—are also simply phenomena arising and departing. Who is the One who witnesses this?

Something very interesting happens when we seek the person we have assumed is somehow located in the body-mind. We cannot find them. We find only sensations and perceptions rising and falling. We find only thoughts emerging and dissolving.

From where do they arise and emerge? Into what do they fall and dissolve?

When we return to our direct experience, we find that every thought, every sensation, and every perception we have ever had arises out of nothing. Such a mystery. We cannot find that from which it emerges, as there is nothing to find. Try it. Try to find the place your last thought arose from. Look into the mirror and see if you can find the place from which the seeing of your image comes.

Why do thoughts emerge? Where do sensations and perceptions arise from? We cannot know.

None of this can be known. For something to be known, there needs to be both a known object and a knower. There needs to be a separation. But there is no separation, though this is how it comes to feel for at least part of our human lives. This is not something to know but something to *be*. It is not possible, in fact, for us to be anything else.

What I am pointing to here is the end of the belief that the body is our identity. This may be painful for thoughts to hear. Thoughts are very invested in separation. Thoughts work hard, day and night, to keep the sense of separation alive. *I am this, I am that, I am the other. I am fat, I am thin, I am happy, I am sad, I am not good enough, I will be okay when my skin clears up.* Thoughts are constantly separating everything out into good or bad, wanted or unwanted, and esteemed or feared.

Thoughts are doing what thoughts do. The quality of a bird is to fly, and the quality of thoughts are to divide. It is the nature of thought to polarise and to suggest polarities like *thin is better than fat* or *a young body is better than an old body* based on the messages it receives societally, to ensure our survival. It is happening in body-minds everywhere. It is simply the themes that are different. In one body-mind, the separation may revolve primarily around the physical appearance; in another, the theme might be around money, relationships, career, health, or other things.

All suffering is the sense of a separation from Love, from our true nature. Of course, we cannot be separate from our true nature. But, to the body-mind, that is how it can feel.

So, we make up these stories about the things we 'need' to achieve to be happy, peaceful, or whatever similar notion it might be. We become focused on getting the perfect body, the perfect house, the perfect job, or the spiritual awakening to fill the sense of separation from Love within us. We are not actually seeking the 'perfect' body, house, job, relationship, or whatever it is at all. We are only ever seeking the Love we already are.

Even this is not accurate. How can Love search for itself? It already *is* that. Yet, the seeking journey is the journey we appear to embark on as body-minds. We appear to separate ourselves from Love when we come into a physical body and then to spend every ounce of our energy trying to find it again. However, there is nothing to find and nobody to find it. It is all a myth, a crazy dream.

Love is not something we find or achieve. It is not like that. Love happens and is happening. Love wakes up to itself, although it never actually fell asleep at all.

The search for wholeness in its many possible guises is so compelling because it appears to work... for a while. When I was about twelve years old, I decided I needed to lose weight. I began to cut out certain food groups and exercise in secret in my bedroom. After a few weeks, I stepped on to the scale in the bathroom and found that the needle had moved down a little. For a moment, as I stood there, looking at the number on the scale, there was a collapse of the seeking energy. There was an incredible soothing of the 'nameless dread' I perpetually carried around with me. I had achieved what I set out to do. I was on my way to becoming more lovable, I thought. A temporary collapse of seeking is often experienced as relief, possibly elation. I felt both very strongly. Then, my thoughts did what it is in their nature to do. They suggested that it was not enough. They suggested that the needle should move down a little further, since I believed I felt neither safe nor lovable yet. And so, I began to topple down a rabbit hole of a depth I could never have imagined.

For some body-minds, it happens a different way. Thoughts profess satisfaction with the new weight but take on another project. Now, to get shinier hair, or whiter teeth, or to tone up a little.

The seeking energy keeps moving on to the next thing—the next number on the scale, the next appearance-focused project—because the sense of separation is still there. The terror of being unlovable is still there.

We do not need to spend our whole lives at the seeming whim of the seeking energy. As Rumi so poetically put it, at some point, we discover that *what we seek is seeking us*. We are not seeking a lower weight, more defined muscles, or whatever it is. We are seeking our very selves.

Falling in Love Meditation

Let us not put this off a moment longer. The time is now and is always now. Now is the moment to fall in love with yourself.

Find a comfortable position, ideally seated with your spine straight, while allowing for the natural curve of the spine. Alternatively, feel free to lie down if this is more comfortable for you. Invite your shoulders to fall down and back away from your ears. Encourage your eyes to become still behind your closed eyelids. Breathe long and deep, inhaling fully and exhaling completely.

Place your awareness on the exhalation in particular. Emphasise the exhale, making it long and active. Notice the short pause at the end of each exhalation before the next inhalation begins.

With each exhalation, have the sense of sinking down into your heart centre. Allow your awareness to 'fall' down into your heart as you breathe out.

As you 'fall' into your heart, fall into the sensations and emotions that present themselves. Fall in love with yourself, deeper and deeper, with each exhalation. Come back into your heart centre. Come back to yourself.

This is your home. They say that home is where your heart is. How true this statement is! Know that you are pure spirit, pure light. Know that you are Love itself and always have been.

Chapter Three

Recognise Appearance-Focused Suffering as an Invitation

Animals do not appear to have a distinct sense of a separate, individuated, personal identity. Rather, they experience life just as that which is arising. The sun comes up and goes down. The tree sways left and then right. The grass appears, is eaten, and then disappears. Just a series of risings and fallings, comings and goings. Just this.

Yet, the animal *does* experience sensing. It is hungry; it eats. It is tired; it sleeps. It moves towards pleasure and away from pain.

The sense of separation we experience as humans—which other mammals do not appear to experience in the same way—is an intrinsic part of being human. The fact that we come to experience our bodies as separate from other bodies is not bad or wrong in any way. It is the natural unfolding of things.

Part of the human experience is to move into the sense of being a separate body-mind. However, a life of subsequent suffering is not fundamental to this sense of separation. Human suffering emerges through the belief that our nature is *the human being as a separate object*, as opposed to our nature being *the knowing of this separation*. Suffering emerges when the body-mind 'forgets' that it is the Beingness itself, as opposed to the object of being.

Our sense of 'I' is our most elementary human experience. There has never been—nor could there ever be—a single moment of our lives within which our beingness, our 'I-Am-ness', was experienced as arriving or departing. The 'I' is not something we are able to witness an absence of. To witness its absence, there would have to be a separate 'I' present to 'watch' its departure.

In modern society, we often learn that the body—which is an

object of our awareness—is who we are. We also frequently learn that the body is partially (and sometimes largely) there to fulfil the needs of others. It is the experience of many children that their bodies exist to express and accomplish the needs of their parents or caregivers and/or exist for their parents' or caregivers' pleasure. Infants and children very commonly learn that an element of the existence of their body is to communicate a certain view of their parents or caregivers to the rest of the world. They are also often tangentially told that they have control over their body, while a large amount of control is exerted on their body from the outside.

We express our distress through the body. How else would we express it? Early in our life, we have a limited repertoire with which to communicate this distress. We retain our faeces or urinate when it is not socially acceptable to do so, we refuse to eat, we vomit up what we have eaten, and all manner of other variations on these things. Such expressive behaviours may become a particularly distinct possibility if we have not been permitted to express our emotions in a safe way: To cry, scream, be ill-tempered, and so on. As we grow into adults, we might find other ways of communicating our distress through the body. Yet, some of us remain stuck in foundational methods related to eating and expulsion of the food that has been eaten. Disordered eating is one colour of this.

More usually than not, the role of our body was decided, to differing degrees, before we were born. Perhaps even before we are conceived. We can also say that it was decided, to some degree, before our *parents* were conceived, or before the conception of their parents, ad infinitum. Certainly, our parents and caregivers may have had very clear ideas about what the bodies of their babies were to be for, prior, even, to conception: For looking after, for holding, for loving, for being loved by, for living out unfulfilled dreams, for being beautiful or 'cute', for showing to others, for providing a sense of purpose in life, for feeding, for putting into sweet clothes, for giving affection to, for getting affection from, for bringing the caregiver company and comfort in old age, and so on.

In the 'good enough' infant-caregiver relationship, there is also room for what the body of the baby spontaneously is, does, and becomes. There is room for the crying, rejecting, vomiting, biting, excreting, or whatever might instinctively emerge. If there is not room for such things, the infant may quickly learn that it is safer to hide these aspects of their bodily experience away, to repress them, or to feel ashamed of them. The arm that might have reached out becomes the arm that stays by the infant's side (impulse without movement). It is likely that this impulse will remain stored in the body as energy that never fired, energy that becomes contracted, energy waiting for an opportunity to be expelled, to tell its story.

So, too, is the mother's body a vessel of creation imbued with needs and expectations long before the infant is born. At conception, and often also during the planning of conception, a whole new set of rules, responsibilities, and expectations may take hold in relation to the mother's body. The mother may see her role (and, indeed, have a notion of this role being thrust upon her) as one of keeping the growing foetus safe and nourished within her. Perhaps she sleeps in certain positions, eats in certain ways, undertakes specific physical exercises to reduce stress and possible physical injury, ingests vitamin supplements, and so on. Her body may become the primary focus not only of her own attention, but also of many other people around her. Suddenly, her body may seem to become the property not only of her partner—if she has one—but also of her family, her community, and the world at large. Overnight, it becomes socially acceptable for complete strangers to put their hand on the woman's abdomen, to ask if she is being sure to refrain from drinking alcohol, for example, and to ask when she is due (and, therefore, when she last had sexual intercourse or was inseminated).

The private body thus becomes the public body. How far this publicisation of the body will go in affecting the mother's view of the body of her baby will be different in each circumstance. It could also be that the body of the baby physically and visibly depletes the body of the mother. It is not uncommon for pregnant women and new mothers to lose hair and teeth, gain weight in unwanted places, acquire stretch marks, lose buoyancy in the breasts and buttocks, and so on. These physical changes may— consciously or unconsciously—play into the mother's opinions and felt-experience of the infant's body, which itself may emerge as unblemished, smooth, and supple—the very aspects of her physical appearance the mother may have 'lost'.

The baby's body is designed by Mother Nature to be captivating and alluring. However pure our intentions may be as parents and caregivers, there is little getting away from the fact that the bodies of our offspring are felt to exist, at the very least in part, for our pleasure. We typically revel in the smell of a newborn baby's hair, the sight of their tiny fingers and toes, the sound of their gentle cooing, and the way their eyes follow us around the room. Even more than this, their existence declares *our own* existence, in no uncertain terms. There is incredible power in the notion that this infant body could not have emerged and survived without the existence of our own body.

Intercorporeality describes the way in which we share and extend our bodily experience. As such, our sense of embodiment is never a private affair. Rather, it is always mediated by our interactions with the bodies of others. Our emotions also occur in this mediated embodiment. Before language and sophisticated thinking, the infant must rely largely on bodily resonance and on their intuitive understanding of others' emotions in their embodied engagement with them. We continue to feel, process, and make sense of emotions primarily within our embodied engagement with others throughout our lives.

Conceptualisations of embodiment are many. I particularly like the thinking of French phenomenologist Gabriel Marcel. Marcel heavily criticised Descartes' conception of the human person, which is perhaps most aptly captured by Descartes' phrase, '*I think; therefore, I am.*' Marcel's understanding of embodiment was that it is not simply a piece of information among other data but is, rather, the absolute starting point and fundamental basis of any human experience or reflection. Therefore, knowing and investigating what it is to be human is not the same as the knowing and investigating of other objects. If we reflect only on the body as an objective 'thing', we miss the concrete experience of the body and the silent 'talk' of the body. This concrete experience of the body is where our essence is rooted for the duration of our earthly existence. We could say, *I embody the body.* Yet, this still begs the question of, *who is this 'I'?*

Life is unfolding. That is our experience. The moment an organic object manifests, it begins to die. The body is certainly no exception to this. Everything is waltzing towards a death. Everything is preceding a transmutation, a transfiguration. The thoughts and the body we like to call 'mine' are not immune to this. Each night, when we fall asleep, we 'practise' falling into this nothingness, into death. The experience of falling asleep is typically not unpleasant or frightening. It is simply a relinquishment of a sense of a personal body-mind living this life, residing in this body, and having these thoughts.

According to many psychologists and psychoanalysts, this sense of disappearing and entering nothingness is the ultimate horror of the human condition. It is the experience the body-mind seems to most deeply dread. Child psychotherapist, Frances Tustin, described this falling into nothingness as a *black hole*, akin to the black holes discovered by astrophysicists some years later. The experience is one of losing our edges as seeming person. It is the experience of being absorbed by a void, of total annihilation.

The sense of impending annihilation had been my terrifying companion for many years prior to alighting the path of self-starvation and self-destruction. I spent half my time feeling as though 'I' did not exist and the other half experiencing the sense of losing the edges of this 'I' to a darkness I could neither control nor understand. It felt as though I was being sucked into a void and was hurtling through the black hole Tustin writes so stirringly about. Thought made two suggestions: I could attempt to escape from the black hole by creating my own reality as a distraction and a shield against the nothingness, or I could try to control my fall into it. In many ways, I ended up doing both. I created my own world in which food was not needed and the usual, innate desire for nourishment was tossed aside. Then, I carefully and meticulously layered control over this pseudo-reality, entering annihilation seemingly on my own terms.

I wanted to be loved and to be a person who was capable of loving others. I believed that my body said, *this is Nicole.* If it was small and thin, it said, *Nicole is non-threatening. Nicole is in control. Nicole is safe. Nicole can be noticed and loved because she is a good girl; she is not greedy and is, therefore, a lovable human being.* I tangentially neglected the felt sense of my body, perhaps in part because I could hardly connect with it.

Creation does not happen within a vacuum (within the body and thoughts of one seemingly separate body-mind). Rather, we create our meanings and notions of reality in our relationships with others. The lives of others, both literally and figuratively, give birth to our own lives. There was a kind of birthing of my objectified body that happened in a continuous creation loop with my mother's conceptualisation of her body... and *her* mother's bodily conceptualisation before her... and so on. The captivating paintings created by Escher from 1916 onwards were an attempt to enlighten the viewer to this truth—that life gives birth to itself in a never-ending cycle, in much the same way as the people in the Escher painting, *Ascending and Descending*, ascend and descend flights of stairs in an infinite loop. I had made all sorts of meanings out of my body as this loop perpetuated: My body as ugly, my body as a measure of my supposed badness, my body as a monstrosity too hideous for another to lay their eyes upon.

I, as a body-mind, held on to my objectified body in order not to 'lose my self', while, at the same time, not understanding who this self was. The loss of the personal identity is terrifying to the body-mind but not to Awareness, which is who we truly are. The loss of the personal identity, in fact, is exactly what a great many religions and spiritual traditions extol. Jesus tells us that we must lose our lives in order to find them. Zen teaches that while it is the clay that forms the pot, it is the emptiness inside that holds all we desire.

Jesus died on the cross and rose from the dead three days later. Guru Nanak went down into the river and his friends feared that he had drowned. Instead, he was in a divine trance in the presence of God, returning three days later to sing God's praises to the world. The Egyptian God, Osiris, was murdered by his brother before being both reborn in the form of his son, Horus, and becoming the King of the Afterlife. Then we have the resurrection stories of Krishna, Ganesha, Dionysus, Attis, and many others besides.

Rebirth is one of the most basic and essential archetypes. The pattern of birth, life, death, and rebirth (*Sa, Ta, Na, Ma*) in religion, mythology, and literature involves a struggle that leads to a new realisation of the Self. This rebirth usually happens because of the trials a figure or character endures. This may be a physical re-birth or it may be a re-birth while in the same physical body. This is the Hero's Journey written about by mythologist Joseph Campbell and others. It is the mesmeric understanding that the 'death' of the false self enables the felt sense of the true Self to emerge.

Could it be that our struggles, whether appearance-focused

or otherwise, are heralds to the archetypal rebirth? Is it possible that the black holes in our lives are inviting us to remember our true nature and to emerge into a life beyond our wildest imaginings?

Let us entertain these possibilities as we proceed through this narrative together.

All is Love Meditation

Find a comfortable seated position (or you can lie down if you prefer), inviting your shoulders down away from your ears and straightening your spine, while allowing for the natural curve of the spine. Have a sense of the base of your spine rooting down into the seat/earth and the top of your spine reaching up through the crown of the head to the sky.

Close your eyes and rub the palms of your hands together vigorously in front of the heart centre for thirty seconds or so. Place the palms over your closed eyes, pressing them gently into the eye sockets. Feel the warmth seeping from your palms into your eyes and take a moment to become accustomed to the intensified darkness.

Breathe long and deep, inviting the sensation of dropping into the darkness. Have a sense of the darkness coming towards you on each inhalation and moving backwards slightly on each exhalation.

Continue to breathe long and deep for a few minutes, sinking your awareness into the darkness surrounding you. Feel into any sensations and emotions that emerge without judgement. If your attention is distracted by thoughts or other phenomena, gently take it by the hand and lead it back to the darkness and to the breath.

Take a long, full exhalation, drawing the breath all the way down to the base of your spine. At the top of the inhale, place your hands on your lap and open your eyes very wide—as wide as you dare. Lightly suspend the breath as you feel fully into the sensation of the light flooding in. Say aloud, with full conviction, *'The light is Love.'* When the impulse to exhale becomes strong, tightly close the eyes, replace the palms over the eye sockets and exhale. As you do so, drop down into the darkness. Say aloud, *'The darkness is Love.'* Notice the pause at the end of the exhalation before the inhalation begins. Again, at the top of the inhale, remove your hands, open your eyes very wide and repeat, *'The light is Love.'* Repeat this cycle for as many rounds as you feel moved to do so. Take time after your practice to sit in silence for a few minutes with the eyes closed, allowing any sensations and emotions to work their way up and out through the body and your deeper being.

Chapter Four

Welcome Your Emotions

In an ideal world, as infants, we would have had the experience of our emotions being taken in by our caregivers, digested, and offered back to us in a more palatable form. We would have had the experience not only of our emotions being *allowed*, but also *welcomed*.

It can be difficult, if not almost impossible, for caregivers to take in their infant's emotions if they were not permitted to feel and express their own emotions when they were young (and if they have not processed and assimilated these early experiences). Current life events can also feed into this, such as mental health issues, traumas, and relationship difficulties.

As we have explored, the infant will do everything in their power to attune to their primary caregiver(s). They will cut themselves off from their interoceptive signals if they must, thereby numbing their emotions. They will amend their expressive behaviour to keep their caregiver(s) close. They will become a false Self to maintain a relational connection.

Infants who have learned to cut themselves off from their interoceptive signals may grow up into children, adolescents, and adults who are not in touch with their emotions. They may feel numb a lot of the time, or they may try to dampen painful, seemingly overwhelming emotions through substances, food, behaviours, and so on. They may have a conscious or unconscious sense that their emotions are dangerous and must be hidden away from others, regardless of the personal cost.

When we boil it down, moving beyond our appearance-focused identity struggles is no more complicated than welcoming, feeling, embracing, and assimilating our emotions. However, 'uncomplicated' does not necessarily mean 'easy', of course. We go to such great lengths to avoid feeling these emotions because we are wired to resist pain and to attempt to keep ourselves safe. On a really basic level, we avoid feeling these emotions because it ignites a great deal of fear and pain to do so.

Survival suggests, *wear a smile, because your tears and your anger will only repel others.* It also asserts, *if you allow yourself to feel sad, you will cry forever and lose yourself in your tears.* So, we put on a brave face and swallow the lump in our throat. *I'm okay,* we say, with our words and our behaviour. *I am the sort of happy, balanced person you will want to be around. I won't frighten you off with my anger/sadness/jealousy/shame etc. Please stay close to me.*

One of the deepest myths pervading current society is that human beings cannot handle their emotions. We are told this explicitly and implicitly, often throughout our lives. We are also fed the message that other people cannot handle our emotions either. So, we become stuck in the frightened/frightening position. We become terrified not only of *our* emotional pain, but also the emotional pain of others.

The fear underlying a great many of our fears is the root fear of not being loved; the fear of emotional and psychological obliteration. Yet, of course, our emotions have never demolished us. If they had, we wouldn't be here to read these words. Emotions do not have arms to strangle us, nor guns to shoot us. Somehow, we have always survived our emotions, however painful they might have been.

Our brain, nervous system, and entire physiology does not know the difference between, *Mummy will not bring me my milk if I show my anger (and, therefore, I will die), my partner will no longer fancy me if I put on weight (and, therefore, I will die),* and *the lion is running towards me (and, therefore, I will die).* Unconsciously, we believe it is all going to kill us. It is all a massive fight for survival. To survive, we need to be cared for—initially, by our caregiver(s), and later, by ourselves. Yet, if we have never experienced 'good enough' caregiving, we will not possess an internal template for self-care. We may, therefore, need to build this internal template up for ourselves.

To survive, the body-mind also believes that it needs to belong. The primitive brain has the sense that there is safety in numbers. So, we hide our emotions from our 'tribe' and try to look like the other members of our community and society in order to belong with them. This is not at all helped by the fact that over 90% of the images we are bombarded with on a daily basis show a largely homogenous body-type, with *beauty=love* being the master narrative. We desperately try to 'fit in', so as not to be exiled and left alone for the elements to ravage us and the lions to eat us.

The primitive brain is working very hard to keep us safe. Its lack of ability to discriminate can put us into a large amount of bother in modern society. We are no longer likely to die if we do not belong to a particular group. But, try telling the brain that!

We can 'teach' the brain that we are safe, actually, to a certain extent. Many of the exercises and meditations offered in this book aim to support you in doing just that. We are likely to continue to be vigilant towards potential dangers, which is a good thing. However, we can certainly become more discriminatory in terms of what we react to and how this reaction unfolds.

It is also possible to learn, both cognitively and somatically, that our emotions are not dangerous. They are not a threat to our survival, but *champions* of our survival. We cannot learn this by telling ourselves it is so, or by reading books like this one. The invitation is to dive into our emotions without reserve. There may be fear. There may be resistance. It is important to remember that this fear and resistance are also yearning for our welcoming embrace.

It can be most helpful to be proactive in this endeavour, as opposed to reactionary. We could practise feeling the emotions as they come up in our day-to-day lives, but this may be more difficult to do in the thick of the triggering event, especially if we don't have an internal template for how to go about this. The first step often seems to be to practise feeling our emotions outside of triggering events. Another piece of this puzzle is that there are likely to be a lot of emotions stuck in the body from the past. Feeling, releasing, and assimilating these emotions will facilitate more space for fresh emotions to emerge and to be processed in the moment, as opposed to being stored and continuing to knock on the doors of our hearts in a bid for resolution.

For some time now, I have had a daily morning practice, a personal *sadhana*. I rise early in the morning and practise some Kundalini yoga and chanting for between thirty minutes to an hour (examples of Kundalini chants are given in Appendix Three and on my YouTube channel: www.youtube.com/c/PointofLight). Then, I sit. I sit and welcome any emotions that may be there. I feel deeply into my body, noticing any resistance or fear, and feel into that also. Sometimes, I sit for some time before I notice anything, but more commonly, strong emotions come up rapidly (or at least, they certainly did in the early days of this practice). I do not try to 'work out' the feelings in my body with my thoughts or make any assumptions about them. Instead, I stay with the sensations that are arising, whatever they might be and however painful they may seem. I open my arms— sometimes, in my mind's eye, and sometimes, in actuality—and embrace any arising emotions like vulnerable children who have been ignored and rejected. For the first few weeks of engaging in this practice, I sobbed for extended periods of time. I learned to go to bed earlier and get up earlier to leave more time for this practice, setting a timer so that I wouldn't need to keep checking the clock if I knew I had to be out of the house for work. I gave my somatic experience my full and unadulterated attention.

I feared that I would be an 'emotional wreck' for the rest of the day after such a practice. I thought I would never be able to stop crying, or I would lose my mind with the pain of it all. This has never been my experience. Rather, this practice leaves me with a sense of relief, release, and openness. Having liberated the body from so much stored contraction, I am more present to the experience of both myself and others as I go about my day. It feels as though a black cloud has been lifted. Feelings of 'nameless dread' are less likely to emerge. Sometimes, more tears do come during the day and these are welcomed also. There is nothing as natural as tears. Then, later that day or the following morning, I return to my yoga mat to give full attention to the sensations underlying those tears.

Sometimes, I also cry through the yoga and the chanting. Or I laugh. Occasionally, I have screamed. And danced. Whatever happens is permitted to happen. A lot can be worked through during mindful movement and chanting. When we chant, we stimulate the eighty-four meridian points in the mouth, allowing thought patterns, beliefs, constructs, and emotions to surface, process, and clear. It is as though the words of the chants are waves clearing through the emotional rubble. As Yogi Bhajan poetically put it, 'What we vibrate, we become.' Beautifully, when sound reaches a certain frequency, it turns into light.

Sometimes, memories will emerge, both procedural (body-based) and cognitive. Let them come. These memories might hurt you or shock you. Welcome and feel into the sensations of pain and shock. You will find that, at a certain point, these sensations will reach a crescendo and pop like a balloon.

All humans experience the same emotions. They might be pinned on to different things, but their substance is the same. You can take the water out of the ocean and put it into different vessels, but it is still all ocean water. The fear in me is the fear in you. The shame in me is the shame in you. The joy in me is the joy in you.

We might be surprised by what we discover when we listen to our emotions as though they are vulnerable, rejected children. We may find that the potential impact we can have on others is a common theme woven into the deepest fears underlying our most repressed emotions. This might be as historic as our fear that our crying would 'kill' Mummy as infants, which makes tremendous sense in the context of the infant's experience of the 'good' and 'bad' objects (please see Chapter Five for more about this). We keep Mummy alive—and therefore, we keep ourselves alive—by stifling our cries and being whatever Mummy needs us to be so that she can be emotionally stable herself. This 'game' starts incredibly young, within the first hour of our lives. Imagine carrying that kind of internal template through your whole life. A great many of us do.

The invitation is to go to the very knife-edge of our pain, ignoring whatever logic might tell us. A much deeper logic is operating here. This is not logic we can describe or negate but can only experience.

When we have created a new internal template—a new somatic understanding that our emotions are not dangerous and will not kill us—we are far more likely to halt any resistance to our emotions in its tracks. We are far more likely to experience a sense of safety within our bodies, feeling the emotions as they rise up and allowing them to tell their story as we watch them assimilate or depart.

In turn, we are also far less likely to feel the need to engage in resistance-based behaviours to suppress or 'manage' our emotions. We are far less likely to overeat or under-eat, over-exercise, pick at our skin, spend hours researching cosmetic surgery, and so on in order to handle our anxiety, to feel safe and to believe we can survive.

The more time we spend with our emotions the more clearly we can come to feel the distinction between these emotions and the One who is aware of emotions. We can begin to have a deeper sense of ourselves as the open, peaceful space of Love into which all emotions arise and dissolve. This does not position these emotions at a distance from who we are. Quite the opposite. It places them as close to our essential essence as all phenomena are, which themselves are made of Love: Closer than close. The difference is that there is no pain in the body that is sobbing, for example, from this place. There are bodily sensations and emotions. There is sobbing. All of this is welcomed and experienced as taking place within the space of Awareness, of Love. The true Self is the space of love into which all phenomena arise and depart. The body-mind grieves and releases in this space. You are this space of Love. Know this, and you will know you are already at peace. You are already free.

'There is no cloud in a cloud,' as spiritual teacher Mooji puts it. And there is nobody in a body. There are bodies, there is sensation, there is perception... and there is the witness to all of this. You are the Witness. You are the one who notices your belly. You are not your belly. You are the one who perceives the wrinkles on your forehead. You are not your wrinkles.

It is the body-mind that suffers. The true Self never suffers at all. There can be physical pain and emotional pain and they can feel terribly real. But *you* do not suffer. You are the freedom itself.

Ask yourself if freedom can suffer. Close your eyes and really feel into this question. If you believe yourself to be separate from freedom, suspend this belief and imagine that you *are* freedom. Is suffering a possibility at all?

I so often hear people talking about feeling choked by numerous possibilities. When there is a battle against the physical appearance, this can manifest as feeling paralysed when choosing which foods to eat, which cosmetics to buy, what diet or steroid pills to take, which cosmetic surgeon to go to, or which clothes to wear. There is tremendous freedom in the notion that, at the level of the body-mind, there is no choosing. Even the impulse to move a part of the body is present for at least half a second before we are consciously aware of the impulse. Our freedom is not at the level of the body-mind. Our freedom is at the level of pure beingness, which is who we truly are.

I remember watching a recording of one of spiritual teacher Mooji's satsangs that really made me smile. He describes stripping the body away, bit by bit. The skin, gone. The hair, the lungs, the kidneys, the heart, gone. He continues until there is nothing left of the body. Nothing at all. He asks, in his cheeky way, *'Is this too gruesome for you?!'* Then, he continues. The mind, gone. The imagination, gone. Memories, gone. Desires, gone. So, he continues, metaphorically stripping away everything we have ever thought comprises a part of who we are. What is left? Try it. Drop everything. Your body, your thoughts, your imagination, your memory, even your emotions. Let it all go. What is it that remains? Find that. That is who you are.

The One who is left does not identify with the body. It does not identify with anything at all. To that One, the body is simply a phenomenon arising in the same way that all objects, sensations, and perceptions arise. The body is no more personal than a tree, a sunset, a droplet of water, or a bluebird. For a while, it may feel closer than other phenomena, as though the body is somehow closer to 'you' than the tree outside your window. The body is perceived as being 'here' and the tree is perceived as being over 'there'. You seem, perhaps, to perceive the tree from your body. It appears this way because that is the way most of us have been conditioned. As we have explored, this was not our experience as infants. Our earliest human experience was a wash of sensations and perceptions. The tree outside our nursery window was as intimate to us as our big toe. Closer than close.

If you return to your current experience, you will find that any object in the room or outdoor area you currently find yourself in is no further away from your awareness (and therefore from you) than your body is. Take any objective phenomena in your present-moment awareness. It might be a solid object, like this book, or it could be a sound, perhaps, or a smell. I am now looking at the glass of water on the table in front of me. I have learnt it is at a distance from me and I need to somehow reach out to get it. But who is this 'I' who reaches? The body reaches out, but from where does the glass and the reaching arise? Where is my experience of it? My only experience of it is my awareness of it. My awareness of the glass arises in the same manner as the awareness of my body and in the same place (if we can call it that). The body and the glass both arise as perceptions within awareness. This awareness is closer-than-close.

Find the one who controls your inhalation and exhalation. Find the one who conducts the beating of your heart. Find the one who raises your blood pressure when you are frustrated and lowers your blood sugar level when you run. Find the one who reaches for the glass. Where is that one? Can you find them? It is the nature of the glass to be still (although, quantum physics tells us that even the glass is in constant movement) and it is the nature of the body to move. When the body is thirsty or bored, it will reach for the glass. Who is the one who observes that reaching? Is that one any more involved with the body than it is with the waxing and waning of the moon?

One of the facets of this story that most seems to cause many of us—particularly those of us in the Western world—so much pain is the notion that we have control over the shape and form of the body. This is in no small part because society has told us our bodies need to look a certain way to be deemed 'beautiful', and that beauty is a prerequisite for being loved. We suffer because we have forgotten (or, so it seems; we never really forget) we are Love itself. So, our thoughts take on board these notions of how we can become lovable. Being thin (if we are women) or muscular (if we are men) are just two examples of that. And so, thoughts arise that if we lose weight, get slimmer arms, achieve a flatter stomach, or obtain a six-pack, we will be loveable and happy. We pin our lovability and our happiness—not to mention our peace, self-worth, hope, and all manner of other things—on to changing the physical appearance of our bodies.

In the beginning, it can feel exciting and tantalising. *I am going to lose ten pounds and others will look at me with adulation. I will have more self-confidence. I will be loved.* And so, we chase, and we chase. Perhaps we lose ten pounds. Yet, somehow, our dissatisfaction with ourselves and our lives remains.

I tried all sorts of things as a child to make myself lovable, although I didn't consciously know this was what I was doing at the time. I tried getting the best grades at school but that didn't seem to work. I tried being the consummate 'good girl' who never displayed any anger or opposition. That didn't seem to work either. I was running out of options to 'make myself lovable'. I unconsciously scanned my environment, looking for some clues. I was young, perhaps ten or so, when I started scanning a bit further afield and noticed a distinctive pattern in what I saw. The suggestion seemed to be—and it was a very loud and clear suggestion—that I could make myself more lovable by becoming thin. Thinness was what all the women around me seemed to want, and what all the successful women I saw in the media seemed to have. Thoughts naturally arose from this new information. Thoughts like, *I should only eat this and that. I must become smaller. If I lose weight, then perhaps I will be loved.* The unconscious backdrop of these thoughts was the foundational human template that love=survival. The body-mind will do everything it can to survive. Ensuring that it is lovable and maintaining a close connection with others is a significant part of this.

The attempt to make ourselves lovable is the *fawn* in *fight, flight, freeze, or fawn*. To *fawn* is to act servilely, to put one's needs aside for another's. Those of us who fawn seek safety and the experience of being loved by merging with the wishes, needs, and demands of others. I am yet to meet a person who struggles with appearance-focused identity struggles like BDD and eating disorders who does not do this to some degree. They tend to behave as though they (unconsciously) believe the cost of any relationship is the total relinquishment of all their needs, preferences, rights, and boundaries. They have usually learned that they must always be compliant to gain and maintain attachments with those around them. They typically struggle to assert themselves or state their boundaries, whether physical, emotional, or otherwise. When they *do* try to assert a boundary or state a preference, they often experience overwhelming flashbacks to infancy/childhood emotions. These are usually unconscious and may not come with any explicit, concrete memory, image, or thought attached to them. Rather, there will typically be a lived sense of the body as being unsafe in the form of an implicit, procedural (sensation-/body-based) memory. The person is likely, therefore, to retract; thus, cutting themselves off from their knowledge of, and ability to express, their needs and desires.

Trauma therapist Pete Walker describes three common subsets of the fawn-type: The fawn-fight type, who coercively or manipulatively takes care of others, smothering them into conforming with their view of whom others should be; the fawn-flight type, who obsessively makes themselves useful to others; and the fawn-freeze type, who numbingly surrenders themselves to scapegoating— the classic domestic violence victim or similar. In my clinical experience, people who end up with diagnoses like eating disorders and BDD tend to have had a relationship in early infanthood—usually with a primary caregiver—of the fawn-fight variety and are most likely to be of the fawn-flight type or a combination of the fawn-flight and fawn-freeze subtypes. I am not suggesting this will be the case for everyone. However, a clear pattern has emerged in my clinical work and personal liaisons which I find difficult to brush aside as attributable to chance. It also feels to be of no coincidence that many people with these diagnoses are of high intelligence and tend to do well academically, later, having a propensity towards workaholism. This is another face, perhaps, of their incessant desire and drive to please.

A growing body of research points to the higher levels of trauma in the histories of those engaged in appearance-focused identity struggles. For example, people with diagnoses of eating disorders and BDD have been found to have had higher levels of exposure to a broad range of risk factors, including childhood adversity and abuse. Strong links between post-traumatic stress disorder and bulimia have been found.

Emotional neglect and abuse have been somewhat more difficult to define, and therefore study, within scientific literature. It has been suggested by some that an invalidating environment in childhood might underlie all forms of relational trauma, resulting in poor distress tolerance and increasing the likelihood of using self-injurious behaviours (including destructive eating behaviours) to manage emotions. Early case reports and studies of family interactions by Minuchin, the father of family therapy, demonstrated that families with a member diagnosed with an eating disorder are more commonly enmeshed, intrusive, and negating of the person's emotional needs. More recent research has found that attachment processes are often fraught in eating disordered populations, with insecure attachment of different forms being common in this group. Insecure attachment patterns are also more common among people diagnosed with BDD than among the general population.

People diagnosed with eating disorders regularly describe a critical family environment featuring coercive parenting. People diagnosed with bulimia often report greater parental intrusiveness; specifically, maternal invasion of privacy, jealously, competition, and paternal seductiveness. Conversely, parental encouragement of autonomy is associated with less-restrictive eating behaviour.

It is clear from the research that trauma typically has some implication in the development of appearance-focused identity struggles for many people. This trauma most commonly tends to have happened repeatedly in the context of a caregiving relationship over time in the person's early life; thus, constituting what is increasingly being referred to as 'developmental' or 'complex' trauma.

There can be developmental differences in children who have experienced complex trauma in relation to self-regulation, planning, working memory, self-reflection, concentration, behavioural inhibition, and many difficulties in interpersonal functioning. People who have experienced trauma who are later exposed to frightening images tend to show extreme arousal in primitive brain regions (such as the amygdala), a deactivation of the brain regions for thinking, and little capacity to inhibit strong emotions or translate feelings into words. Thus, it may be that when people ask us why we hate our bodies so much, we cannot find an answer to offer them. Similarly, we may not be able to wrap words around why we starve, overeat, or harm ourselves. This is because the 'reasons', if you will, are not stored in the cortical part of the brain, nor in the left side of the brain—both of which are tasked, broadly speaking, with reasoning and logic. Rather, they are embedded in our primitive and limbic brain and in the right side of our brain, which are sensation-based and embedded within implicit, stored emotions.

Complex trauma generally reduces the experiencer's ability to use their bodily reactions and emotions for guidance about what is, and what is not, safe. In this way, the body of an infant/child who has been exposed to complex trauma can become wired to act quickly to survive any potential danger. The sympathetic (fight, flight, freeze, fawn) nervous system may go into overdrive, or parasympathetic (rest, digest, freeze, fawn) activity may become heightened, or we may come to oscillate uncomfortably between the two. As we have already touched upon in the first chapter, another possible line of defence is the activation of the dorsal vagal system—we learn to dissociate and disconnect not only from our own emotions and bodily sensations but also from the world around us.

Complex trauma typically causes changes in the brain's circulatory and hormonal systems. These can become embedded patterns over time. The high levels of stress experienced by children exposed to developmental trauma means they are likely to grow up with higher cortisol levels and altered brain organisation. Indeed, research has shown that people diagnosed with eating disorders typically have altered cortisol regulation in comparison to those who have not received this diagnosis. Other studies have shown that trauma and stress can adversely affect rewards systems in the brain, within which dopamine is centrally implicated. This can significantly diminish enjoyment of life and engender fear in relation to social contact, which are only two examples of possible ramifications.

The experience of developmental trauma, therefore, can alter the lived experience of our bodies mechanistically. This might cause a person to feel 'stuck' in, for example, their overeating or self-starvation behaviours. Yet, it does not have to be this way.

The interface between biological processes and awareness is a fascinating one. The smallest unit of matter (a quark) behaves differently depending on whether it is being observed. If you put a quark under a microscope and observed it, it would behave like a particle. When unobserved, however, it would behave like a wave. Matter is directed by — or, one could say, imbued with — awareness. Matter is not divorceable from awareness since it is a modulation of awareness. The biological mechanisms of our body-minds, therefore, are modulations of awareness also.

The experience of developmental trauma can impact the way our brain and nervous system develop. However, our brains continue to be malleable and neuroplastic across our lifespan. In addition to this wonderful truth is the fact that, of course, both the developmental trauma and the resultant biological mechanisms are, themselves, modulations of awareness.

I can take the example of my self-starvation behaviours. I

starved myself, in part, to soothe my nervous system, which had become entrenched in an oscillation between heightened sympathetic arousal and parasympathetic arousal due to my early life experiences. Each time I tried to stop starving myself, I felt overwhelmed by feelings of nervous system arousal and panic. Thus, I would return to self-starvation to feel numb and to soothe myself. I felt totally stuck in this cycle. At a certain point, I wanted to stop starving myself but felt like I couldn't face the bodily sensations that arose when I did.

In many ways, I felt trapped by my biology, never mind the emotional aspects of my self-starvation (of course, both were irrevocably intertwined). The sense of *I am trapped* whirled around constantly in my thoughts. At a certain point, I became fascinated by the question of who the 'I' was whom I had taken myself to be. I began to ask myself, *Who is this "I" who is trapped?* I began to delve into this question, as though it was the most important question in the world.

I began to become fascinated by who I truly was. Who was this 'I' who felt a lack of freedom? Who was this 'I' who felt numb when my body was starving? Who was this 'I' who felt unlovable? When I returned to my direct experience, I could find the panic and numbness as physical sensations arising in my awareness, but I could not find a personal entity who was suffering on their account. There was a witnessing presence of the bodily sensations, but there was no sensation of suffering in this witnessing presence. What I had been calling 'suffering' was simply the bodily sensations arising and dissolving in this space of awareness, which my thoughts then attached themselves to and labelled. When I felt into the bodily sensations of panic, a racing heartbeat, tightness in the chest, and shallow breathing etc., without resistance I found that there was no suffering. And the sensations, having told their story, departed as swiftly as they had arrived.

Over time, my nervous system has learned to react less and

less virulently to perceived threats in the environment. The conditioning has gradually been updated. This reduction has taken considerable time and has been helped greatly by yoga and other mindful movement practices, which we explore in more depth in Chapter Six and Appendix Three. Indeed, it can take a long period of time for the body to play out the consequences of its conditioning and release any trapped trauma and emotional pain. This process is nothing to be afraid of. This, too, is a modulation of our essential nature, a modulation of Love.

The psychological and physiological ramifications of developmental trauma emerge in our essential essence and can dissolve in our essential essence. They perpetuate because we turn our gaze away from them, because we shove the frightening sensations and thoughts away with overeating, starvation, repeatedly gazing in the mirror, and all sorts of other behaviours. Each time we experience a frightening sensation in the body or a seemingly unbearable thought, we are being drawn into a portal of healing. Each of these sensations is an invitation to feel the underlying emotions we were unable (for whatever reason) to feel at the time of a past trauma, and to fully assimilate the experience. This is not only important but necessary for the body-mind's sense of safety, peace, and wholeness.

I hope the following exercise will support you in the commencement of your process of welcoming, feeling, and assimilating your stored emotions.

Sending an Invitation to your Repressed Emotions

Find a comfortable seated position with paper and a pen nearby. Take a few moments to notice the sensation of your breath coming into and out of your body. Notice your breath without judgement, without trying to change anything about it at all. As you breathe, you may notice movement in parts of your body; perhaps in your chest area, abdomen, or back. Or you may notice no movement at all. That is fine. These are all just possibilities. The simple invitation here is to direct your awareness towards your breath. If you notice any resistance as you place your awareness on your breath, welcome this without judgement, allowing it to be there just as it is.

Try, if you can, to locate the movement of your diaphragm as you breathe. As you breathe in, your diaphragm moves down, allowing your lungs to fill with air. As you breathe out, your diaphragm moves upwards, pushing the air out of your lungs. You might like to place your hands, fingers spread, on and above your navel to get a sense of this.

Recall how the diaphragm and chest area are one of the emotions' favourite hiding places. Say 'Hello' to the emotions hiding out there in whichever way feels spontaneously natural for you to do so.

Take up your pen and paper and write, 'Dear Emotions,' at the top. Maintain a connection to the sensations in the area of your diaphragm as you do this. Continue by writing a letter to your emotions, inviting them to begin to reveal themselves to you over the coming weeks and months. Your letter might go something like this:

Dear Emotions,

Thank you for holding my story. Thank you for refusing to depart until the experiences of my life in this body have been borne witness to and assimilated. Thank you for refusing to leave, no matter how hard I have tried to push you away. I know you are the portal to my healing and am sorry I have avoided you for so long.

I am ready to start hearing my story; to start feeling all you are here to allow me to feel. Please be patient with me. I may need to go slowly. I have a lot of fear that you will hurt me and that I will get lost in you forever if I entertain you. I am gradually understanding that this is both myth and avoidance but I seem to go in and out of this understanding at the current time.

I have put aside half an hour each morning for us to spend time together. This is our special time and I will give you my full attention during this period. Your part of the deal is to show up and my part of the deal is to feel and express whatever emerges. I know you will visit *at other times in the day also, but I want to give you a designated space to tell all the stories I was unable to feel and hear at the time they occurred.*

Thank you for your patience and your understanding. Let us begin. You are my dear friends and I love you,

Nicole x

Take time after writing your letter to be kind and compassionate to yourself. Nurture yourself in a sensory way, perhaps through a hot bath, a hug, a walk through nature, or whatever you feel will be imbued with the most self-compassion and self-love.

Chapter Five

Heal Your Relationship with Food

Physical sensations are part of our biology. Physical sensations, such as hunger, are totally natural. We are born with the ability to sense our hunger. This interoceptive signal exists to ensure that we get our needs met and to ensure our survival.

Whilst totally natural — necessary, even — hunger is something that many human beings come to have a hard time with. All sorts of things can become attached to this hunger: Denial, greed, neediness, danger, fear... the list of possibilities is endless. The sensation of feeling hungry and the deed of eating can morph into something very far from the basic act. How does this come to be? And can we ever escape the topsy-turvy relationship with food so many of us come to know?

The clue, perhaps, is in the idiom I used in the last sentence: Our *relationship* with food. When we look at it closely, we find that food, just as everything else for the body-mind, comes back to relationships, to love.

The act of taking food into the body is one of our earliest relational experiences. We cannot obtain food for ourselves when we are infants. We must wait for the breast or the bottle to come to us.

Psychoanalyst Melanie Klein believed the first gratification an infant receives from the external world is the satisfaction experienced from being fed. Feeding, therefore, becomes the prototype — the template if you will — for all internal and external experiences with the object world. Klein believed the most obvious relationship symbolised by food is that of the mother, the one who provides this food. In short, food comes to symbolise the child's relationship with their mother/primary caregiver:

Food = Mother
Mother = Food

It can happen that the symbol becomes confused with the object. Food becomes confused with the mother.

In typical development, the infant has an emerging awareness of differentiation and separation between the body-mind-self and other objects. The infant can separate themselves from the mother if they feel safe and contained enough to do so.

At first, the infant is postulated by Klein and others to split the objects in their environment—of which the mother is one— into either 'ideally good' or 'wholly bad' objects. This splitting happens since the infant is not yet able to conceptualise two possibilities simultaneously, such as an object having both good and bad aspects. As a result, the infant only sees 'part objects'— it sees the 'all good' or the 'all bad' in every object they perceive.

To keep themselves safe, the infant aims for a total union with the 'good' objects and a total annihilation of the 'bad' objects, as well as a total annihilation of the 'bad' parts of the body-mind-self. Any 'bad' object that is perceived to threaten the 'good' object is feared with a dread beyond imagining—a *nameless dread,*' as psychoanalyst Wilfred Bion referred to it.

As we explored in Chapter One, the infant is entirely dependent on the primary caregiver for their survival. Any experience of their emotional needs failing to be recognised and attended to can be a trauma for the infant. Since the infant is only developmentally able to view objects as either 'all good' or 'all bad', the infant is unable to counterbalance any 'badness' with the goodness it earlier received from the same caregiver. Therefore, the infant whose needs regularly go unmet is in a near-constant state of terror.

It is important to add that young infants have not yet achieved the developmental stage of object permanence. They do not yet understand that an absent object can return, such as a mother who is out of sight. This adds to the fear they experience. When we consider that the infant absolutely needs the primary caregiver for their survival, we can perhaps understand how utterly terrifying the thought of the departure of the caregiver, or the notion that they are 'all bad', can be for the infant.

To soothe their terrors, the infant employs certain defences, which allow them to keep the 'all good' and 'all bad' experiences separate. At the same time, they attempt to acquire the attributes of the good object, expel the bad qualities, and avoid separation. Whatever the cost.

For the infant to separate the body-mind-self from the caregiver, the infant must be able to integrate 'good' and 'bad' to some degree. All 'good' and 'bad' aspects of the self must be recognised as part of one body-mind-self. Only once this implicit understanding takes place can the body-mind-self and the caregiver be experienced as separate body-minds. Absolutely necessary to this process is the notion that the infant has enough goodness inside them and that there is enough goodness in the caregiver. There must have been sufficient 'good' experiences so that there is enough 'good' to withstand the 'bad'.

Infants who are unable to separate from their primary caregiver often remain 'stuck'; in part, due to their unconscious fear that their 'badness' will destroy both their caregiver and themselves. What may then emerge is a striving to contain, and ideally, stamp out, the supposed badness.

Since 'food' and 'caregiver' are intertwined for the infant, food can organically become a symbol for the caregiver, as opposed to feeding being experienced as one of the caregiver's functions. A fusion is simultaneously experienced between the body-mind-self and the caregiver. Food becomes the symbol within which this fusion is felt and, therefore, rejected.

Put very simply, the infant who experiences the body-mind-self as 'all bad' at the start of the process of individuation (or at any time during this process) needs to protect the caregiver from themselves if both are to survive. Thus, food is rejected as a symbolic rejection of fusion with the caregiver. This occurs since a direct rejection of the caregiver would mean total annihilation of the relationship, and therefore, annihilation of both the caregiver and the body-mind-self.

The way we take in food and expel it speaks volumes about our early caregiving relationship. The infant who cannot separate themselves from their caregiver may come to reject food in a symbolic act of rejecting fusion with the caregiver. They may later replicate this and end up with a diagnosis like anorexia. The infant who experiences a high level of ambiguity around whether it is safer to keep the caregiver close or separate from them may come to both take in and reject food simultaneously. They may later replicate this and end up with a diagnosis like bulimia. Another possibility is the infant who experiences an intense lack of fusion and comes to consume food in large volumes to 'consume' the caregiver and become one with them. They may later replicate this and end up with a diagnosis like binge-eating disorder.

Mary Ainsworth's attachment styles seem to map on to these patterns very clearly. The avoidant-attachment pattern often springs from infantile experiences of the avoidance of emotions. It may have been that the primary caregiver, for whatever reason, was not in contact with their emotions and/or found the emotions of their infant to be overwhelming and frightening. (This is not to attribute blame in any singular direction. We know the biggest predictor of a mother's attachment pattern with her infant is her infantile attachment pattern with her own mother. These experiences are transgenerational, and we often fail to look 'far enough up the river' when we are responding to behaviours like self-starvation, purging, and so on. Typically, caregivers do the best they can at the time, given their experiences and emotional resources. We must step outside of the 'blame the other' culture we are living in in order to truly heal, while tangentially acknowledging each facet of our story.) The relational template for the infant who experienced an avoidant-attachment style with their primary caregiver is likely to include cutting themselves off from their own emotions. Interoceptive sensations like hunger will also likely be denied, due to the fear the associated expressive behaviours ignite in the caregiver. This can set up a pattern of avoiding emotions, neediness, desire, hunger, food, and so on. Diagnoses like anorexia and orthorexia may then emerge later as metaphors, expressions, and modulations of these experiences. As the person avoids and rejects food, they avoid and reject emotions alongside rejection of the sense of abandonment and fusion with the caregiver themselves.

Children whose earliest attachment patterns are anxious or ambivalent have usually had mixed caregiving experiences. Their primary caregiver may have been attuned and emotionally available sometimes but not always. The resultant sense for the infant is one of unpredictability. The infant is confused. *Sometimes Mummy responds to my cries and sometimes she does not. Sometimes Daddy holds me tenderly but sometimes he hurts me.* The relational template is likely to involve confusion over whether to pull the caregiver close or push them away, and whether to take food in or push it out. This may result in binge-purge types of behaviours and diagnoses like bulimia and binge-eating disorder. It may result in a person oscillating between different diagnoses, mirroring the confusion they experienced in their early lives.

Infants for whom their earliest attachment relationships have been disorganised are likely to have experienced some form of abuse and/or neglect. They may have had the experience of being treated as the 'bad object', no matter how very hard they tried to be good. The relational template is likely to involve a strong pull towards harming the self in the most unthinkable ways possible, perhaps through self-injurious behaviours like drinking corrosive substances alongside disordered eating behaviours in the context of food and body image struggles. Suicidal ideation and suicide attempts may be tragically common (though they can, of course, occur across all forms of attachment patterns). Food may be rejected as a metaphor for both rejection of the caregiver and also the 'bad self' or may be consumed in large amounts (particularly, unpalatable foods or non-food items) in a desperate bid to consume the caregiver (or abuser) and in an unconscious bid to literally become their caregiver as opposed to being their victim. The taking in of large quantities of food may also be an unconscious attempt to make the body itself 'unpalatable' to the abuser.

There is a transitional space between 'not-me' and 'not the other'; a space between fusion with the caregiver and the sense of a separate body-self. To move from complete fusion to individuation, infants use what Donald Winnicott called 'transitional objects'. For many infants, these objects take the form of soft toys, a blanket, a thumb, and so on. The transitional object allows the infant to have a sensation of soothing the self without the presence of the caregiver.

In appearance-focused identity struggles, the objectified body itself would appear to become the transitional object. The infant failed to arrive at a sense of a boundary between the body-mind-self and the caregiver and, thus, the transitional space was not maintained. The infant has the experience of continued fusion with the caregiver, perhaps into adolescence and possibly even beyond this.

Food can become imbued with all sorts of terrifying meanings, such as the fear of losing the other and the fear losing the self. In this way, a reluctance to eat food or to keep food inside the body can be a means of starving off a threat and keeping away the unbearable feelings projected on to an infant (and later a child and adult) by the caregiver.

My own history is a clear example of some of these processes. While weaning in infancy, I became very selective about which foods I would and wouldn't eat. My mother took me to the doctors on more than one occasion because I would only eat eggs for long stretches of time and nothing else. Food became a battleground between myself and my mother from a very early age. I rejected what she offered me and ate only what my infant mind had assessed permissible. Unconsciously, it seems to be that I was playing out our insecure, enmeshed relationship through my rejection of food. My infant self was unable to separate in any way from the intense fusion between myself and my mother, so I did the only thing that was within my power to do. I rejected the food as a symbol of my rejection of the self-mother fusion. I would come to repeat this pattern many years later in the form of a diagnosis of anorexia, with catastrophic ramifications.

Interestingly, when my parents divorced some years later, I found myself repeatedly eating uncontrollably in the middle of the night. Shortly after my mother left the family home, I began what I now understand to have been a desperate attempt to consume her. I consumed and consumed and consumed until I could take in no more. And yet, I still felt utterly empty inside.

Later, as my relationship with my mother began to heal, I found myself able to eat typical quantities of food with less guilt and without overfilling my stomach. I stopped bingeing in the middle of the night also. As I separated from my mother and rediscovered my own personhood, I began to rediscover my hunger signals and to eat foods, for the first time in many years, which I experienced as satisfying and nourishing. At a certain point, food became food, as opposed to the symbol of my enmeshment with my mother and, therefore, something I needed to be afraid of, reject, or stuff myself with.

Many people who engage in appearance-focused identity battles appear to struggle with separation and individuation. This struggle most typically stems from their earliest caregiving relationships. In many ways, the lack of a sense of edges of the body-mind can be likened to the experience of the infant who has no sense of separation. The difference is a matter of identity. Whilst the infant does not ascribe an identity to the edgeless phenomena, the person engaged in an appearance-focused identity battle suffers because they yearn to be connected to others *as* a separate self. Thus, fusion and separation are sought after simultaneously.

This confusion between the need to separate and the desire to remain fused with the primary caregiver is symbolised through confusion with food. Should the food be eaten or not? Is the food 'all good' or 'all bad' (a position we often see in the diagnosis of orthorexia)? Is the food needed or is it possible to survive without it? The other part of this story is, of course, that if the desire (such as the desire for food) does not exist, then the mother does not need, unconsciously, to exist either.

A necessary element of repairing a pained relationship with food, therefore, would appear to be an acknowledgement of the meaning that food holds. If food does indeed represent our earliest relationship(s), it can help tremendously to figure out what our methods of eating and expelling food are communicating about these relationships. This can support us in assimilating any unresolved emotional pain and healing these relationships, whether with the other person/people or in the privacy of our minds and hearts.

The invitation is to return our pain to where it belongs—to our relationships with others and with ourselves, as opposed to a projection of this pain on to the food we do or do not eat and/ or on to the appearance of the body. The invitation is to look beyond our seeming fear of putting on weight, or of eating or not eating certain foods and explore what is *behind* this fear. If we search earnestly, we will find that these surface-level fears are always rooted in the fear of not being loved.

Just as food can symbolise our relationships with others, so, too, can our relationships with others symbolise our relationship with ourselves. We fear and reject the seeming 'badness' in others because we fear and reject the seeming 'badness' in ourselves. Diagnoses such as anorexia play this projection out in a very particular way. The hypothesised 'badness' in the self is felt keenly and rejected through self-starvation. Tangentially, the seeming 'badness' in the other is too painful to acknowledge and the notion of punishing the other is unbearable. The punishment, therefore, falls on the body-mind-self—with the body-mind-self symbolising the body-mind of the other. Thus, the other is punished by proxy. The mother must watch on as the body of her son withers away. The father must bear witness to his daughter's refusal of the food she needs to keep her body alive.

As infants, each time we took in a meal, we literally took in our caregiver, since we had no notion of separation between ourselves, the food, and the provider of the food. We do not lose this foundational template until we have emotionally separated from our caregiver. Rather, we continue to have the unconscious sense of taking our caregiver in when we eat, although we almost certainly do not consciously conceptualise it in this way. If we cannot separate from our caregiver for whatever reason (if individuation is not possible as infants and children) we may become stuck, in an emotional sense, in the oral stage of development, when we are completely dependent on our caregiver(s). The way we relate to food can thence play out the rejection of the enmeshment. We refuse to take in both the caregiver and the food. We force a separation by forcing the food, which is synonymous with the caregiver, to stay or to be expelled outside of ourselves. Or we stuff ourselves with food in a pained attempt to take the caregiver in.

Each time we eat, we experience the very same response of fulfilment and nurturance we experienced as an infant. For some of us, this sense of fulfilment can be excruciating. It can remind us of the unconscious pain associated with our early attachment relationships or it can be totally outside of our experience if we rarely felt fulfilment as an infant. For others, there can be a sense of being unable to achieve this fulfilment, no matter how much food is taken in.

It is never too late to individuate and separate from our primary caregiver(s). We can do this whether we are two years old, twenty-two years old, or ninety-two years old. We can do this whether our primary caregiver is alive or has died, whether they are willing to make this journey with us, and whether anyone external to ourselves changes their behaviour towards us or their perception of us in any way. We can separate and individuate in the privacy of our own minds and bodies by welcoming, feeling, and fully embracing any emotions that are waiting to be assimilated and by remembering who we truly are. When we release and incorporate the pain of our past into our wholeness, we find that there is no sense of identity embedded in the act of eating or not eating. We no longer need to avoid, compulsively take in, or expel our primary caregiver, and so, we no longer need to avoid, compulsively take in, or expel our food. The emotions which narrate that part of our existence have told their story. Totally naturally, the denial of food and overfilling ourselves with food will then drop away.

Looking Further Up the River

You may have come across the parable of the river. It goes something like this:

One night, villagers were sitting by their riverbank, about to eat, when one villager noticed a young child floating upside-down and drifting down the river. Several villagers jumped to their feet, dived in, and tried to rescue the child. It was too late.

A short while later, another young child was noticed, coughing and screaming as it struggled to stay afloat. This time, the villagers were luckier and the child, although bruised and battered, lived.

This turn of events continued and the frequency with which the villagers had to attempt to rescue children from the river increased.

Sometimes, the villagers were successful, but this was not always guaranteed.

Soon, the resources and manpower of the village were directed at saving as many children as they could. This activity occupied the villagers constantly and other endeavours they had previously pursued were forgotten, but this was accepted, as it was a worthy cause.

One day, two villagers began to walk away from the village, heading upstream. They were questioned, 'Where are you going?! We need you here.' The villagers replied, 'We're going upstream to find out why these children end up in the river.'

Food and body image struggles do not emerge in a vacuum. They are a symptom of something deeper. The clue is to be found further up the river, not solely through the presentation of the person and their seemingly personal distress.

Creating a Family Tree/Genogram

Creating a family tree or genogram can be an excellent way of exploring further up the river. It is helpful to include as much rich information in this family tree as you can. Explain to your family members that you are creating an information-rich family tree and would like to hear more about your grandmother, great-grandmother, great-great-uncle, and so on. Try to ask questions that reach beneath the surface level. Some ideas might be:

- *'What was it like to be brought up by your mother?'*
- *'If your grandfather were still alive, what do you think he would say about his role as a father to your mother?'*
- *'What would Auntie say about what it was like to have Grandpa as her father?'*
- *'What was the relationship like between your mother and father? What do you think your mother and father would say about their relationship if I asked them?'*

- *'What did your mother/father see the role of children as being?'*
- *'Was anyone on your side of the family ever treated for psychological struggles or mental illness, as far as you know?'*
- *'Have there been any tragedies on your side of the family?'*
- *'Have there been any early deaths on your side of the family?'*
- *'Has there ever been any talk of abuse or neglect on your side of the family?'*
- *'What was it like for you growing up?'*
- *'Did you feel loved growing up? Tell me more about this.'*
- *'What are the happiest memories of your childhood?'*
- *'What caused you to feel most afraid during your childhood?'*
- *'What was going on with you in your life at the age of [insert age]?' (This is good question to ask your mother or father if they are still alive, using the age when you first started struggling with food and body image issues. You can ask your grandparents also.)*
- *'What have been the biggest struggles in your life? What has brought you the most heartache?'*
- *'If you could change one thing about your childhood, what would it be?'*

It can be helpful to use photographs for your discussion, as they can be excellent visual prompters for memories. They can also reveal implicit aspects and give you further avenues for questioning. For example, *'You look like you are hiding behind your brother in that picture, Nan. Do you remember what you might have been feeling at the time?'*

From the information we have gathered, we can begin to create a picture of what childhood was like for our parents and grandparents. We may be able to begin to make links between our own attachment experiences and those of our parents. As we have explored, attachment patterns are very often transgenerational—literally, 'passed down' from one generation to the next. Though, of course, as soon as we are aware of such patterns, we can opt to break the pattern and parent our own children—if having children is a part of our story—in entirely different ways.

The nuances of transgenerational attachment patterns are likely to be unconscious. They will typically be stored in the implicit memory, and therefore, not easily captured by conversation alone. We will not fully 'get to the bottom' of our parents' and their parents' attachment histories by spreading out the family photographs and asking a range of questions. But it is a very good place to start and can be incredibly illuminating. You might also like to conduct further exploration through researching online and in archives. There are even some companies who will trace your family tree for you.

Family therapy can also be incredibly helpful in terms of looking further up the river and should, in my opinion, be the absolute mainstay of any clinical treatment for food and body image struggles. Similarly, some of the exercises in Chapter Eight may support the creation of a deeper connection with your relatives, which may subsequently engender greater ease of conversation and sharing. It may also support the individuation process if this still needs to happen.

Chapter Six

Come Back into Your Window of Tolerance

Physical sensations are the theatre of our emotions. It is through the sensations of our bodies that we both connect with and individuate from our caregivers. As we began to explore in the last chapter, it is never too late to find our own edges and to relate to our caregivers outside of an enmeshed state.

We try to escape the physical sensations and the emotions in our body because we have the sense that they are too much for us to cope with. We believe that we feel overwhelmed and terrified by our emotions, and so we escape into the behaviours we have used to help us feel safe over the years.

When our emotions are responded to in a 'good enough' way, we can stay within our window of tolerance. Professor of psychiatry Dan Siegel proposed the Window of Tolerance model, describing how exposure to threat or trauma stimulates the autonomic nervous system, resulting in sympathetic and parasympathetic hyper- and hypo-arousal states. When the threat is over or has been removed, many infants (and children and adults) continue to suffer from autonomic sensitivity to stimuli, whether directly or indirectly related to the traumatic event or events. The person can come to experience a confusing array of physiological, emotional, and cognitive 'symptoms', including over-reactivity of the stress-response system and negative beliefs about the self. People often describe (and/ or express through their behaviour) that they struggle to tolerate emotional and physiological states without becoming overwhelmed. In the context of appearance-focused identity struggles, the person may turn to food (such as overeating or under-eating), to mirror gazing, to trying to 'fix' an aspect of the appearance etc. to negate this sense of being overwhelmed and in an attempt to bring the self back into the window of tolerance.

Dan Siegel proposes that there is a 'window'—a range of optimal arousal states within which emotions can be experienced as tolerable and experiences can be integrated—between the extremes of hypo- and hyper-arousal.

Window of Tolerance

Hyper-arousal Zone	**2. Sympathetic 'Fight or Flight' Response** Increased sensations, flooded. Emotional reactivity, hypervigilant. Intrusive imagery, flashbacks. Disorganised cognitive processing.
Window of Tolerance Optimal Arousal Zone	**1. Ventral Vagal 'Social Engagement' Response** State within which emotions can be tolerated and information integrated.
Hypo-arousal Zone	**3. Dorsal Vagal 'Immobilisation' Response** Relative absence of sensation. Numbing of emotions. Disabled cognitive processing. Reduced physical movement.

Figure One: The Window of Tolerance

As infants, the attunement of our primary caregivers would have enabled us to stay within, and return to, our window of tolerance. For example, we may have experienced hunger that took us momentarily outside our window of tolerance. We may have then demonstrated this through our expressive behaviour, such as through crying. If all worked out well, our caregiver would have heard and understood our cry, provided us with milk, and we would have returned to our window of tolerance. If such attunement was frequently absent, we may have found ourselves suspended outside our window of tolerance for extended periods of time. As we have already explored, many of us would have coped with this by disconnecting from our interoceptive signals. Of course, the pangs of unmet hunger are less likely to be distressing if we cannot feel them. So, too, are the unmet needs to be touched, to be witnessed, to have our emotions digested and offered back to us in a more palatable form, and to be loved.

It is possible that infants who learn to cut themselves off from their interoceptive signals may grow into children (and possibly, later, adults) who spend a significant amount of time outside their window of tolerance. This can become their 'norm' both emotionally and physiologically. As children and adults, we have more means at our disposal for attempting to get ourselves back into our window of tolerance in comparison to the infant, who cannot move much, communicate verbally and so on. The list of possible ways we attempt to soothe ourselves and bring ourselves back into our window of tolerance is as long as the universe is wide. Food is one obvious way and can be compelling, due to its innate links with nurturance and the sense of a met need. It *is* typically comforting to fill our bellies with food. Yet, someone inside their window of tolerance tends to stop eating when their body is satiated. If we are hyper-aroused or hypo-aroused, we might continue to eat beyond this point, and to keep eating until we have a sense of being soothed (of coming back into our window of tolerance). Similarly, we might try to starve or over-exercise ourselves back into our window.

Rather than using food, over-exercise etc. to soothe ourselves, we can engage in other, more true-Self-serving behaviours.

71

I have found the behaviours linked to our early attachment experiences to be particularly beneficial. These behaviours also give us a 'second chance' to rewire the brain and psyche, to have a sense of security in our bodies, and to trust our emotions, and thus, to individuate from our caregivers if we have remained enmeshed with them.

The rest of this chapter contains only some of many possible suggestions for bringing yourself back into your window of tolerance. Some yoga postures and practices are mentioned. If you are interested in finding out more about these postures and the broader practice of yoga, please see the Further Reading List for some excellent texts on the subject. Yoga centres and classes can be located through the Yoga Alliance Directory (www.yogaalliance.org/Directory), the Kundalini Yoga Teachers Association (www.kundaliniyoga.org.uk/class-finder) and by conducting a local Internet search. Yoga Therapists can be located through the International Association of Yoga Therapists (www.iayt.org/page/MemberSchoolOverview) and the British Council for Yoga Therapy (www.bcyt.co.uk/bcyt-members.php).

It is important to highlight that the practice of the postures of yoga is concerned neither with flexibility nor physical exercise. It is not the movement itself, but the attention we bring to the movement which transforms the postures into yoga, particularly the attention we bring to the breath. As we move in synchronicity with the breath so we create a moving meditation; thus connecting to spirit and to our true Selves.

There are many forms of yoga and I would highly recommend trying different disciplines out to find a practice best suited to you and your needs. Some forms of yoga are more calming and promote the activity of the parasympathetic nervous system, while others are highly stimulating and ignite sympathetic arousal. I have personally found that Kundalini yoga—the *Yoga of Awareness* as it is often referred to—most effectively and efficiently connects me to my true Self. On a physiological level, my body revels in the repetitive, stimulating practices of Kundalini and the balance of my nervous system is thereby achieved, often in very short spaces of time. Kundalini yoga as taught by Yogi Bhajan has a vast range of Kriyas (sequences of movements/exercises/practices) for encouraging both sympathetic and parasympathetic nervous system stimulation depending on what your needs are at any given time. Meditations are also offered for just about everything including a vast array that encourage the feeling and assimilation of emotions and sensation-based experiences in the body.

Yielding

Yielding describes our relationship to space and gravity. In part, it describes the way the infant learns to feel the weight of their body relax into the ground as it is supported by the external environment. Later, the infant will learn to yield their weight into their arms and legs to facilitate crawling, followed by yielding into the legs for walking. The infant needs to feel safe enough to 'let go' to do this. Resistance to gravity creates rigidity in the body or the feeling of being overtaken and defeated by the gravitational force.

Some practices we could explore to return to this part of our developmental trajectory and bring ourselves back into our window of tolerance might include:

- Yielding yoga asanas (e.g., forward folds, child's pose, pigeon, supported fish, reclined butterfly, and corpse pose). Yin yoga can be particularly good for this. Most yoga asanas are, in fact, yielding postures, if practised correctly
- Thai yoga
- Bundle rolls from the practice of Kundalini Yoga
- Lying on 'sinking' or moving surfaces without rigidity (e.g., waterbeds, beanbags, sand, soft mud, and snow)

- Yielding the weight into less common parts of the body (e.g., elbow platform)
- Being carried or held by another

Overcoming Gravity

Before the infant is born, they have explored a variety of postures in utero. According to yogic philosophy, the infant has undertaken a total of eighty-four postures in the womb, which directly map on to the eighty-four core yoga asanas in Hatha yoga. Between fourteen and sixteen weeks gestation, large body movements peak, such as whole-body flexion and extension, stretching, and leg-kicks. It is not until after birth, however, that a strong experience of gravity comes into play. The infant develops by managing increasingly erect postures over an increasingly small base of support. This typically happens top-down, from their head down to their feet.

The infant's struggle to overcome gravity supports social interaction. As the baby becomes able to hold their head up, for example, they have more opportunities for initiating eye contact with their primary caregivers and others. In the context of a 'good enough' caregiving relationship, gratification emerges from these initiations. A lack of gratification is likely to take the infant outside their window of tolerance.

Returning to our struggle against gravity as adults can soothe and heal current emotional experiences and reactions related to these earlier experiences. Some examples are:

- Yoga. Most asanas work against gravity in some way. It can be helpful to mimic the developmental trajectory by starting with asanas that work against gravity in relation to the head, then moving down through each body part, to the toes. For example:
  - *Head: Camel pose, wheel, handstand, peaceful warrior, triangle, and revolved triangle*

- *Torso:* Bridge, headstand, handstand, crow, wheel, and peacock
- *Arms:* Half-moon, warrior poses, chair, stretch pose
- *Hips:* Warrior two, bridge, pigeon, butterfly, camel, cow-face, wide-legged forward fold, and dancer
- *Legs and feet:* Shoulder-stand, handstand, boat, Kundalini lotus, stretch pose, locust, and bow
- Running, skipping, walking, and dancing
- Jumping (such as on a trampoline)
- Swinging
- Cycling
- Sports (including team sports)

Dynamic Postural Control

Our bodies are always in motion, even while we are sleeping. Similarly, some sitting and standing postures may appear to be stationary but involve the body gently swaying back and forth on its base of support. This sway gives us proprioceptive feedback which tells us where our bodies are in time and space, and enables us to maintain our balance. This maintenance of balance would have fed into our attachment behaviours as infants; for example, allowing us to reach out with our arms to be held and to remain upright in order to be seen more easily.

Behaviours and exercises that explore our postural control can, therefore, be tremendously healing. Some of these include:

- Yoga and other mindful movement practices (such as Qigong, Tai Chi, and mindful dance)
- Alexander Technique
- Feldenkrais Method
- Sensorimotor Psychotherapy
- Rosen Method
- Rolfing

Reaching, Pulling and Grasping

Reaching, pulling and grasping are core ways in which we explore and interact with our environment as infants, and a key means by which we build a relationship with our primary caregivers. One of the earliest developmental patterns to emerge is the rooting response (reaching with the mouth). The first motor nerves to myelinate, in fact, are the sucking nerves. Being led by their sense of smell, the infant reaches with their mouth in search of the breast or bottle. Once the teat or the nipple has been found, the infant grasps on to it and begins to suck in rhythmic bursts. The sucking action creates a rocking of the upper jaw and the skull on the lower jaw, while the neck muscles shorten and lengthen alternately. The sucking action is a whole-body event, activating the muscles along the back of the body via the spinal column and down the front via the oesophagus.

For some infants, the attachment relationship is such that the reaching-grasping-sucking action does not complete its cycle. Without the necessary support from, and attunement with, their caregiver, the infant struggles to stabilise. They tense their neck and abdomen and may be unable to grasp the nipple effectively. Strain is placed on the muscles and soft tissues of the spinal column and the digestive tube as tension mounts at the base of the neck and in the abdomen. Sensing is reduced and motor coordination is impaired. If this cycle repeats itself on numerous occasions across time, the infant is likely to become uncertain about whether nourishment and comfort will be available to them, thereby further restricting the emergence of a secure attachment with their caregiver. The infant is left hungry, yearning, longing, and dissatisfied. They are also left with stiffness in their spine and digestive tract.

The infant's developmental reach pattern integrates into the nervous system, both reflecting and influencing their whole-body experience. Some ideas for soothing and assimilating any emotional pain related to this part of the attachment history and, thus, bringing one back into the window of tolerance, could include:

- Yoga—Sitali breathing
- Yoga—Ujjayi breath
- Yoga—Whistle breath
- Neck rolls
- Bringing the chin to the chest and holding it there for a few seconds or even minutes while breathing deeply
- Activating the back muscles through yoga asanas (e.g., forward folds, half-moon, cat/cow, Sufi grinds, spinal flexes, Kundalini windmills, triangle, revolved triangle, bridge, cobra, and downward-facing dog)
- Neck and back massage
- Chanting (for some examples of chants, please see Appendix Three) and humming
- Sucking on a thick liquid (e.g., yoghurt or thick smoothies) through a narrow straw
- Eating thick soups, mashed potatoes, and custards
- Chewing on hay, pine resin gum, or similar

Successful contact on reaching for an object with the hands comes after reaching with the mouth. This usually occurs between eleven and twenty-four months of age but reaches at this point are usually jerky and asymmetrical. It takes years before the infant's/child's hand reaches become as smooth as most adults' hand reaches. Having made contact with the object, the infant may then pull the desired object towards them.

Reaching precedes grasping and pulling, as control of the arms precedes control of the hands. Therefore, it may be beneficial to explore reaching movements prior to grasping and pulling movements as adults, should we wish to revisit these attachment-based movements and discover our ability to self-soothe within them. We might like to try:

- Reaching postures in yoga (such as warrior poses, stretch pose, balancing table, chair, twisting lunge, forward bend with shoulder stretch, gate, and wide-stand forward twist)
- Grasping yoga postures (such as seated forward fold [holding on to the legs or feet], bow, dancer, Ashtanga binds, mermaid, Kundalini lotus, extended hand-to-big toe pose, and bear grip)
- Picking tree-fruits
- Painting the ceiling
- Cleaning (e.g., stripping beds, removing cobwebs, and dusting hard-to-reach places)
- Hulling peas, shelling nuts
- Gardening (e.g., dead-heading flowers and pulling up weeds)
- Sewing and other handicrafts

See below 'Learning to Walk (and Pulling)' for other pulling-based practices.

Pushing/Pushing Down

Pushing is the process of pressing the limbs or spine away from a thing or person. This includes pushing the feet into the floor to stand. A push sends a compressive force into the body, organising lines along pathways of movement. This action is crucial for nervous system and brain development during infancy. Some practices that can support a revisiting of this stage of development include:

- Thai yoga
- Yoga asanas that involve a pushing element (e.g., all standing postures, downward-facing dog, balancing half-moon, handstand, crow, and right-angle with feet pressed into the wall)
- Resistance training

- Swimming
- Rowing
- Baking (e.g., kneading dough)
- Hoovering, sweeping, and mopping
- Planting seeds and bulbs
- Pushing a wheelbarrow

Learning to Walk (and Pulling)

The average age for taking the first walking steps is around twelve months, although the age-range can be quite broad (usually between eight and eighteen months). To be able to walk, the infant must have sufficient strength and balance to support the body on one leg as the other leg moves forward. The suggestions given thus far can support an exploration of balance, which can be very beneficial in bringing us back into our window of tolerance. For example, it is amazing how soothing the simple act of standing on one leg can be when we are feeling both hypo- and hyper-aroused. Yoga postures which are also balances include: Eagle, tree, dancer, side-plank, crow, and Kundalini lotus (to name but a few). Some examples of other activities necessitating balance include: Tai Chi, cycling, heel-to-toe walking and walking along a line on the floor.

Learning to crawl and walk maps closely to our attachment as infants. It provides us with a means to move towards our caregivers, and to move away from them if we need to. In the 'good enough' caregiving relationship, the infant actively moves towards their caregiver and receives the attunement and comfort they need. Re-exploring those early walking skills, including pulling yourself up by your arms, can support a return to the window of tolerance through proprioceptive awareness. Proprioception is always soothing and organising for the system, which is why we might find ourselves, for example, swaying or rocking when we feel distressed. Here are some things you might like to try:

- Inviting another person to pull you up by your arms from a seated to a standing position
- Hanging on monkey bars or from a door frame
- Pull-ups
- Aerial yoga
- Rope swing
- Pulling on a piece of anchored rope (or playing tug-of-war!)
- Climbing trees
- Using gymnastic bars
- Swaying back and forth in a standing position
- Walking on less-familiar materials (e.g., mud, sand, clay, or walking through water)
- Walking on tiptoes
- Walking on stilts
- Trying to walk after a period of bouncing on a trampoline
- Mindful walking or walking meditation (i.e., placing your full attention on the act of walking as you move slowly and mindfully—this can be paired with long, deep breathing)
- Falling in a controlled, safe way (e.g., on to a gym mat or a bed)
- Falling and allowing a loved one to catch you (i.e., falling backwards into their arms)

Obstacle Navigation

As infants, we must find our way through and past physical obstacles to reach the arms of our caregiver. We must go around, over, under, and sometimes through objects. This is quite a skill. The infant must select the required movements and modify them accordingly. In the first few weeks after acquiring a new posture, such as crawling or walking, the infant falls repeatedly over what seem to be impossibly steep slopes, high steps, and wide gaps. These falls provide a rich opportunity for attunement and soothing. In the 'good enough' caregiving relationship, the infant's distress is relieved by the voice, touch, and containment of their primary caregiver when they stumble over yet another object in their path. If this regularly fails to happen, the infant is likely to perceive a world full of barriers and dangers from which there is no support or reprieve, catapulting them firmly outside their window of tolerance.

Some ways we can replicate this developmental stage as adults to revisit any associated stored emotions and/or provide soothing for ourselves might include:

- Walking up and down stairs mindfully
- Weaving in and out of objects as you walk (e.g., laying a series of cushions on the floor and walking around them in figure-of-eights, perhaps while listening to some mantras/ soothing music)
- Jumping over objects
- Limbo
- Mazes/labyrinths
- Roller-skating and ice-skating
- Mindful jogging or walking on busy streets and in crowded places
- Mindfully cycling through rocky terrain
- Obstacle courses
- Tai boxing
- Sports (e.g., dodgeball, rugby, hockey, football, and basketball)

Exploring the content of this chapter may have reminded us why movement is so important and can feel so good across our lifespan. It is never too late to revisit early developmental patterns, feel into any associated pain, and literally rewire our brains and nervous systems by re-exploring and perhaps amending some of our early somatic patterning. Some of the suggestions given here might sound very simple. I hear you asking, 'Can sweeping *the kitchen floor really bring me back into my window of tolerance?'* It most certainly can! When undertaken mindfully, with a focus on bodily sensations, it can also be a conduit for procedural memories related to part of your developmental history. So, feel into your body as you sweep; notice how your arms move as you push and pull the broom; experiment with exaggerating the movements and notice what sensations, emotions, and thoughts this brings up for you. Try not to overthink it. Wilfred Bion described the propensity for thinking to be a defence against feeling. Rather, *feel* into the experience of sweeping. Allow any and every reaction to come to the surface, welcoming every sensation with open arms. You might find yourself sweeping long past the point of the kitchen floor being clean. This is more than fine. It was never about the kitchen floor anyway.

Meditation for Using Movement to Come into the Window of Tolerance

Find a comfortable, seated position, with your spine erect while allowing for the natural curve of the spine. Tuck your chin in slightly to bring your spine into a comfortable alignment. First, become aware of the following five-sense perceptions, noticing what you can see, hear, smell, taste, and touch. Second, move your awareness towards the inner sensations of your body, perhaps noticing your breathing, heart rate, any pain or tension, differences in temperature in different parts of your body, and so on.

Now, place your awareness on any movement that might be happening. For example, you may notice the movement of your diaphragm as you breathe or a slight swaying in your body as you sit. Now, direct your focus to your thoughts. Notice your thoughts arising and dissolving, becoming interested in whether the thoughts seem to come and go in a stream or whether they tend to stick around and become more circular. Next, notice any emotions that are alive in your body. Direct your attention towards these emotions, diving into them as deeply as you feel able to do so. Finally, point your attention towards your transcendent sense of Self, the sense of Self beyond the body. Sink into this sense of your true Self and rest there for a little while.

The six aspects we have just explored are the six Organisers in sensorimotor psychotherapy, namely: Five-sense perception, inner-body sensations, movement, thoughts, emotions, and spirituality. These are the six core ways in which human beings organise their experience. The Organiser we found ourselves most easily directing our attention to in the first part of this meditation can offer us some clues as to what Organisers are predominant in our lives; thus, inviting us, perhaps, to develop the others. (See the Further Reading List for more information on sensorimotor psychotherapy.)

For the second part of this meditation, I ask you to think of a thought you would like to endorse in your life related to your experience of eating and/or your physical appearance. For example, you might like to choose a thought such as:

- I have a strong, vibrant body.
- I choose foods that nourish and sustain me.
- I love my stomach.
- I embrace my physical appearance.

Take your time to select a thought that you would like to be true in your life, and say it out loud, with as much conviction as you can muster. As you say this thought aloud, notice where this thought seems to sit in your body. Do you feel it in your chest, arms, feet, pelvic area, head, or somewhere else? Repeat the thought until you become aware of an associated physical sensation in your body. Don't worry if this feels incredibly subtle or if you can only feel it in a tiny area, such as your left little finger. The strength and size of the sensation does not matter. Simply dive into the sensation.

As you immerse yourself in the embodied thought, allow the sensation to begin to extend throughout your body. Permit your body to move in whichever way spontaneously emerges. See if the sensation becomes a gesture or a posture. Extend and exaggerate this gesture or posture, sinking ever more deeply into the sensations that emerge as a result. Remain in this posture for at least thirty seconds, allowing brain chemistry changes to take place. Embody your thought-sensation with every fibre and sinew of your body, 'becoming' the thought in bodily form.

Take a snapshot of your posture or gesture in your mind. Know that you can return to this posture or gesture and, thereby, access the embodied sense of your chosen thought at any time.

Chapter Seven

Recognise That Your Body is Socially Constructed

Human life is made up of relationships. This much is clear. We come into the world completely reliant on our relationship with our primary caregiver for our survival. Many of us then appear to spend the rest of our lives desperately clinging to our relationships with others, terrified of being alone and of not being loved.

There is a whole-body response of utter terror when we have the sense that we are not lovable. We attempt to escape this terror, and come back into our window of tolerance, by trying to make ourselves lovable and by soothing the terror with under-eating, overeating, the use of substances, repetitive sensory behaviours, spending hours researching cosmetic surgery and all sorts of other things.

Human beings are social animals. We are all longing to belong and our lives do not happen in isolation. Rather, it is not unusual, as psychoanalyst Wilfred Bion so affectingly highlighted in his work, for human beings to give up a part of themselves to remain a part of the group. Body-minds believe they need the group to survive.

Our bodies are not bodies in isolation. They are bodies among the bodies of others. Our thoughts are not thoughts in isolation. They are thoughts among the thoughts of others.

Wilfred Bion suggested that groups operate in two conflicting ways based on two distinctive mental states, which he called 'basic-assumption mentality' and 'work-group mentality'. 'Work-group mentality' describes the extent to which the members of a group can manage their shared tensions and anxieties to function effectively. In contrast, 'basic-assumption mentality' describes the state of a group when it is taken over by strong emotions, such as anxiety, fear, hope, guilt, and so on. At the point of operating from a basic-assumption mentality, the group loses touch with its purpose. The result of such a loss of purpose is typically a kind of freezing, a sort of stagnation.

In all groups, there is an ever-present danger of losing part of our self-identity to the crowd-identity. There is typically a constant tension in groups: How much does a body-mind stay true to the authentic self and how much do they attempt to cover up or adapt this self to fit in and remain a part of the group?

The whole is not solely the sum of its parts. Often, the group takes on a 'mind' of its own. Thus, we move from the body-mind to the group-mind. Many of us are members of numerous groups, including family groups, work groups, friendship groups, community groups, cultural groups, and society at large. Most peculiar things can occur within body-minds when they find themselves as part of a group-mind. These peculiarities can become magnified in the context of being a member of numerous group-minds.

Just as we desperately strive to remain attuned to our primary caregiver—both to ensure our physiological survival and because we are intrinsically wired for love—so, too, do we strive to attune to the group for these same reasons. Therefore, it is perhaps not difficult to understand why so many of us attempt to amend the body when the societal mentality is one of beauty being necessary to ensure connection with others and secure experiences of love.

Our bodies are emotional entities. Thus, a group focus on the appearance of the body moves us from a work-group mentality to a basic-assumption mentality. At this point, the group loses touch with its purpose. It stagnates. Currently, society as a group is stuck in the notion of beauty being equitable with lovability. The true purpose of the group—such as to provide support and companionship to its members—is, arguably, increasingly becoming lost.

Many of us are currently living in highly-individualised cultures in the Western world. A core feature of collectivist cultures is that individuals often subordinate their personal goals to the goals of a collective, which is usually a stable in-group, such as a family or tribe. Therefore, the goals of the individual frequently reflect the goals of the family or tribe. In individualist cultures, on the other hand, there are significantly more in-groups, such as co-workers, clubs, and interest groups. Thus, much of the behaviour of the individual is centred around goals that are consistent with these various in-groups, resulting in demands and behaviours which are less stable and more segmented.

In extremely complex individualist cultures, such as those that have emerged in the industrialised Western world, the number of in-groups are much more expansive, resulting in greater independence from others, as well as greater emotional distance from them. Many of us appear to have more social connections than ever before in history, largely because of technological advances, including the Internet and mobile phones. However, we have far fewer genuine social bonds and community-based obligations. In the late 19th century, Émile Durkheim (one of the founding fathers of sociology) gathered data from across Europe to study factors which affected the suicide rate. His clearest finding was that people who had fewer social bonds and obligations were more likely to take their own lives. Durkheim concluded that people need social obligations and constraints to provide structure in, and meaning to, their existence. More than a century of further study has confirmed Durkheim's findings, with social relationships continuing to be the strongest predictor of contentment and lifespan. Such contentment is underpinned by the sense of being an authentic Self among authentic others.

To fit into individualist cultures, we need to constantly amend the selves we project. Such a reshaping of the body-mind self can be a very lonely pursuit indeed. Within current individualist, capitalist societies, we may be bereft of a community to turn to since we are increasingly living further and further geographically from those with whom we have long-standing connections. We may refrain from turning to our parents, since the lives we are now living are somewhat incomprehensible to them, given the rapid increase in life choices and opportunities in recent decades. We may not consider consulting our religious leaders, since most of us are now choosing to live largely secular lives. We can, perhaps, turn to the plethora of self-help literature—the recent boom of which is obvious on bookshop shelves—but still, we must sit alone with these books and try to figure everything out largely by ourselves. Such individualism sets the stage for a unique and unprecedented constellation of loneliness, disconnection, and despair.

Body-minds crave a sense of belonging and a whole host of negative effects can ensue if this belonging is sensed to be lacking in any way. A great many of us in modern Western society come to assimilate the myth that our bodies need to look a certain way to belong to our groups and society at large. Therefore, we come to blame our bodies for our loneliness, our sense of being outside the group or society, and our sense of being unloved.

Individuals diagnosed with eating disorders have been found to frequently lead secret and lonely lives which typically involve emotional separation from family and friends. For example, people who binge-eat frequently isolate themselves to engage in their binge-eating cycles. Feelings of loneliness can also lead to increased food consumption in restrained eaters and a desire to binge in people diagnosed with bulimia. Loneliness has also been found to be a potential factor contributing to relapse in people diagnosed with both bulimia and anorexia. Furthermore, it has been suggested that early experiences of loneliness may contribute to the development of eating disorders. In one study, women with a history of bulimia and anorexia-binge/purge subtype reported more feelings of loneliness as children than other members of the population.

If we feel dissatisfied with our appearance, we may assume others share our negative view and, thus, isolate ourselves to stave off potential ridicule and rejection. Ironically, this can subsequently feed into notions of unworthiness, translating into greater distaste with our physical appearance and further isolation and loneliness. Thus, a vicious cycle is set in motion, which can become self-amplifying.

The shift from traditional mass media to a system of horizontal communication networks centred around the Internet and other forms of wireless communication has catapulted us into a fundamental cultural transformation through the introduction of a multiplicity of communication patterns. Within this cultural shift, new depths of loneliness are arguably provided with fertile conditions for growth. Technology can make human relationships abstract and, therefore, impersonal. The use of the Internet, for example, has been correlated with experiences of social disconnection. While, on the one hand, the Internet allows us to overcome geographical limitations and connect with people all over the world, many researchers have found that Internet usage, being a solitary activity, detracts from the time a person spends interacting on a face-to-face basis with others, and therefore, can be detrimental to authentic connection with others.

On the UCLA Loneliness Scale, one of the questions posed to measure loneliness is, *'How often do you feel that people really understand you?'* Those of us wrapped up in appearance battles rarely feel understood, which is hardly surprising, given the seemingly illogical nature of our behaviours. An outsider might ask, *'Why would a person wish to starve themselves, throw up their food voluntarily, pay for cosmetic surgery after cosmetic surgery, or spend hours lifting weights every day?'* As we move through this book, I hope we can increasingly appreciate that these behaviours are symptoms of deeper, underlying emotional suffering and that better questions to ask would be, *'What has led you to such behaviours? What is your story?'*

Another way in which community support has fallen away in recent decades is via secularisation, which refers to the shift away from religious values and institutions towards non-religious and secular establishments. When modern people decided that the doctrine of the soul was a bit too religious for secular society, the idea of a self came into being. People, then, who once thought of themselves as having an eternal soul now come to think of themselves as having a unique self, with all the qualities that were once attributed to the soul now being attributed to this self. The difference, and perhaps our tipping point, is that the soul was viewed as a collective and pure manifestation of the Divine/Love/God, while the self was depicted as being highly individualised and riddled with contradictions.

Consequently, so many of us in the Western world no longer view our core as being embedded in Love but as being solely located in personal self-efficacy and responsibility. We are told repeatedly that we have the power to control our experiences, that we are responsible for creating 'beautiful' and societally acceptable bodies, and that we are largely accountable for everything that happens to us. This places a huge responsibility on our shoulders. This suggests that everything is our fault. However, the deeper truth is that, *'No man is an island,'* as John Donne once famously put it, and that a significant, if not central, element of the human experience is to reach out to, seek support from, and connect with others.

The prominent American pragmatist, William James, discussed the components of self in his book, *The Principles of Psychology,* published in 1890. James argued that all people who associate with the terms 'I', 'me', and 'mine' can, in some way or another, be associated with an investment of the self to differing degrees. He claimed that the understanding of this self can be separated into three categories:

- Its constituents
- The feelings and emotions aroused (self-feelings)
- The actions prompted (self-seeking and self-preservation)

The first category (the constituents of the self) can then be further sub-divided into:

- The material self
- The social self
- The spiritual self
- The pure ego

The material self, which appears to be the focus of many individualist societies and appearance battles, is constituted by our body, clothes, immediate family, and home. According to James, it is these things that we are most deeply invested in, because of our outlays of self within these things. The more of ourselves we invest in these objects (i.e., the more we identity with them), the more attached we consequently become to them.

The configuration of our social self is based on our interactions with society. We analyse the reactions of others and this contributes to our idea of our social self. Each person seemingly possesses multiple social selves, perhaps altering their behaviour and even their personality according to which social group they are in. In this way, many of us present a range of social masks to a diversity of people and situations.

The spiritual self is said by James to be our most intimate self, the most authentic version of who we think we are and should be. This spiritual self is comprised of our conscience and will.

Finally, James addresses the pure ego. For James, the pure ego is that which provides the thread of continuity between our past, present, and future selves. This continuity gives us a perception of consistent individual identity, which arises from a continual stream of consciousness. According to James, the pure ego, unlike the ego depicted in most New Age literature, is similar to what many of us think of as the soul.

Just as individuals have a pure ego, so, too, does the group have a group-pure ego. Put another way, the seemingly individualised soul is One Soul expressing in different forms. All beings emerge from Oneness, ultimately continue to be a part of this Oneness, and return to the fullness of this Oneness at some point at the end of the cycle of birth, life, death, and rebirth. This Oneness is synonymous with Love.

It appears to be the case that we temporarily forget we are the soul as human beings, pinning our identity on to the body and the mind. This forgetting is part-and-parcel of the human experience. The human experience provides the soul/Awareness/Aliveness/Beingness/Consciousness/Love with the opportunity to know Itself as its true Self. The separation is the conduit through which we remember and know experientially who we are. We do this by *following our bliss,* as mythologist Joseph Campbell so poetically put it. Our bliss is the call of our soul to itself. This bliss is not equitable with happiness necessarily. This bliss most likely will lead us to the very heart of darkness as this is always where the most profound treasures lie.

To follow our bliss is to discover and to live the purpose of our lives. The purpose of our lives is not to fit into a pair of size-eight jeans, have the clearest skin of anyone in our office, or agonise over what to eat, how much to eat, and when we should eat it. The point of life, as Yogi Bhajan put it, is *to be a point of light*. The purpose of our lives is to know ourselves as ourselves, and to remember that we *are* the Freedom; we *are* Love.

Everything in life emerges in cycles and waves. Breathing, pain, exhaustion, hunger, day and night, the existence of the body… everything. Can you point to something in life, aside from pure beingness, that does not come in cycles? Thoughts cycle as well. The thoughts you have today will cycle around, changing form and flavour over time. Thoughts are one of the main ways in which the mythical separation from Love is maintained.

Our thoughts, in fact, are not our thoughts. Consider where your thoughts come from and you will find that your thoughts come from the group-mind and the societal-mind. A thought that says, *'You shouldn't eat that cake; it will make you fat,'* almost certainly came from your culture and society. It might have come via a magazine, the lips of your mother or your peers, an overheard conversation in a café. It surely did not come from your true Self, and therefore, does not 'belong' to you at all. I invite you to try putting your self-deprecating thoughts into the third person: *I am fat* becomes *She is fat*. You might be surprised to note that this 'new voice' reminds you of someone, typically an adult figure from your childhood who held a position of power in your life.

The invitation here is not to get rid of your thoughts. That isn't going to happen! The invitation is not even to fundamentally *change* your thoughts, for that is resistance, and resistance only perpetuates that which is being resisted. Take your stand knowingly as the Love you are, and your thoughts will no longer be personal. When your thoughts are no longer personal, the suffering that appeared to be embedded within them falls away.

Giving Thoughts a Job Description

It is not uncommon to become identified with our thoughts. It is also not uncommon to feel as though our thoughts are 'taking over' and that they are somehow in the driver's seat of our lives. It can feel like the mind is the master and we are the dog.

Thoughts will always strive to be in control as this is what they were designed to do. They are doing their job very well! The invitation is not to hate or berate thoughts for doing the task they were designed to do but to replace all our complexes with the singular complex: *'I am Love'*. When we know that we are pure spirit having a human experience, when we know that we are Love, the mind sinks into the heart and the true Self becomes the master of the body-mind's experience.

Thoughts like to be busy and will always seek something to become busy with. If we leave thoughts to their own devices, they will run roughshod over our lives. The invitation is to give thoughts a task to do; a task that is in alignment with our heart. If the mind is occupied it cannot be preoccupied. It is our freedom and our task to decide what to occupy the mind with.

A primary task of our thoughts is to support our emotions in keeping us safe. They go about this by splitting everything into 'all good' and 'all bad', and trying to convince us that we need to resist, hide from, fight, and escape anything that is potentially a threat, anything that is possibly 'all bad'. The issue is not that our thoughts are trying to keep us safe, but the belief that is placed in the danger they suggest. The issue is that we take our thoughts as truth. As Yogi Bhajan inquired, *'Do you prefer the voice of truth or your own intellect?'*

Let us do as Guru Nanak suggested and put our head in our hands and lead with our hearts. It can be helpful to provide your thoughts with a 'job description', explaining to them how they can best serve your heart and your higher self. An example of such a job description is offered below:

Job Title: Thinking Part of Nicole
Main Purpose and Scope of the Job: *To store and provide practical information. To put into words that which has been understood at a visceral level, when it is useful to do so. To support the emotions in keeping the body-mind safe.*

Position in Wholeness: *To report to the emotions, who will let you know what you need to say. To be directed by the heart. To orientate yourself towards infinity. To pluck the strings of the nadis (the channels through which the prana [divine energy, life, and consciousness] streams).*

Duties and Key Responsibilities: To remember practical information, like the need for Nicole to bring her purse when going to the shops and how she can get home. To inform Nicole of when she needs to carry out practical tasks, such as reminding her of meetings and deadlines. To put sensations and ideas into language when needed for sharing with others and/or solidifying for wholeness.

Duties Outside of your Remit: Rumination, regurgitating what others have said to Nicole in the past, attempting to manage or push down emotions, attempting to stimulate emotions (with all due respect, they manage you, not the other way around), and assuming control of the body-mind's decisions.

Thank you for your role in my life, Thoughts. I'm afraid I can only give you around 5% of my time and attention, as my soul requires at least 95%. You have been given to me to serve my soul and my destiny. I value you and I love you.

I am sure you can think of many additional elements to add into this job description. Have fun with this! The crux of the exercise is the assertion that your thoughts are neither you, nor are they in control of you or your emotions. Put your thoughts into their place, with kindness and compassion.

Yogi Bhajan recommended recording what you say for a whole day and then listening to it in the quiet of the evening (make sure you obtain permission from the people you are speaking to if you decide to do this). Another transformative practice is to speak your thoughts out aloud, record them, and listen to the recording in an open space of awareness. This can be incredibly powerful.

Chapter Eight

Heal Your Attachment Relationships

Infant experiences that fail to be contained, felt, and thought about inevitably result in guilt and shame. Guilt is a separation which can, at least, be thought about. Shame is a more pervasive and damaging form of separation, as it comes with a sense of being unable to repair that which somehow feels to be broken. Shame is often stored in our procedural, implicit memory. We feel it acutely, although we often sense that we cannot quite grasp it or, therefore, do anything about it. It is the deepest form of separation.

Somehow, experiencing a sense of separation is a part of this dance we call life. Every being seems to go through it, despite not being born with a sense of it. Even after the identification with this sense of separation dissipates, sensations of separation in the body usually continue to emerge. It can become another form of seeking to attempt to remove this sense of separation. We can therefore enter many so-called spiritual practices to 'get rid of' the sense that we are a separate body-mind and to split off any sense of guilt and shame. In so doing, we strengthen the sense of separation even more.

The paradox is that, at the truest level, we encompass both the separation and the non-separation. We are all of it. We are both the feeling of contraction and the feeling of expansion in the body. We are both the sense of a person 'over here' and a sense of a non-person, located everywhere. We are both the feelings of fear and the feelings of freedom. The issue is not the sense of separation but the identification with, and resistance of, the sense of separation. When we cease resisting even this sense of separation, the sense that the 'I' is somehow located within it collapses. There is a realisation that the sense of separation *arises* in who you are; it is not who you are.

The witnessing presence of all phenomena, the Awareness we are, is in a constant relationship with all phenomena since all phenomena are made from it. The body is made from awareness. Thus, the body is in a constant relationship with awareness. It is inseparable from other phenomena, despite its seeming edges of skin which define and delineate it. The body would not exist if it was not in a relationship with everything else.

When we directly experience our deep connectedness with all other phenomena, the judgement and persecution of the body slips away, since this is only possible when identification is present. This slipping away may happen overnight or it may, more likely, be a gradual process as years of conditioning gradually work their way up and out, and are assimilated. Very poignantly, this does not happen in isolation since the body does not exist in isolation. As the conditioning unravels from our bodies, we find that our bodies are in a relationship with other bodies, and indeed with other phenomena, and that these relationships shift and transform. This can happen the other way around also. As our relationships with other facets, including other people, in our lives shift, so, too, can our perception of our body shift, particularly where early or current attachment figures are concerned.

We have explored a few practices of delving into the 'I' we have taken ourselves to be and shall continue to do so as we move through this narrative together. This exploration inevitably leads to the 'we', or rather, to the collapse of all 'I's' which brings forth an irrevocable sense of the collective. We will now look at a few exercises for exploring the nature of the body in relationship to other bodies and for finding the 'we' within the 'I' and the awareness within both.

Eye-Gazing

This can be practised both with a person with whom you feel you have a relational connection and with an unknown person. Sit opposite the person at the same eye-level. Set a timer, maybe for three minutes to begin with (this can be built up as you become more comfortable and familiar with the practice). Begin with your eyes closed. Relax your shoulders back and down and lengthen through the spine, while allowing for the natural curve of the spine. Tuck your chin in slightly. Turn your awareness towards your breath. Notice your breath coming in and going out. Place your awareness on the length, tempo, and quality of your breath without judgement. If your thoughts wander to something else, gently bring them back to your breath, perhaps directing your attention specifically towards the sensation of air in your nostrils or the subtle movement of your breastbone.

Next, direct your attention towards any bodily sensations. Place your awareness on any areas of contraction or tension, or perhaps on any body parts that feel relaxed. You might like to scan through your body with your awareness, starting at the tips of your toes and finishing at the crown of your head.

Finally, turn your attention around to Awareness itself; to the one who is aware of your breath and your body. Sink your awareness into the deepest part of yourself. When you attempt to place your awareness on Awareness itself, you may experience a stillness and a collapse of the sense of subject and object. Whatever you experience or do not experience, stay with the intention to direct your attention towards your awareness (to that which is aware of being aware), to your sense of 'I'.

At some point, the timer you set at the beginning of the practice will go off. When this happens, it is time for you and your partner to open your eyes. Open your eyes slowly, taking time for your pupils to adjust to the light. You might like to place the palms of your hands over your eyes, opening your eyes and gradually opening your fingers, allowing the light to seep through. Slide your hands down your face, letting in the full amount of light.

Meet the gaze of the person opposite you, keeping your gaze soft (as though you are looking across the horizon). Remain steeped in the sense of yourself as the witnessing presence of everything that arises and dissolves. As you gaze into the eyes of the person opposite you, notice the witnessing presence that is witnessing you. Behold the very same awareness with which you stare, staring back at you. Feel the connection between you and the seeming other person. Drop all that you have been told about separate people, separate bodies, and separate identities. Sink into the gaze of the other and notice that you are irrevocably connected with them. You are Awareness and they are Awareness. You are Love and they are Love.

White Tantric Yoga

White Tantric yoga comes from the tradition of Kundalini yoga. It involves chanting and engaging in various movement and breathing (pranayama) exercises, mostly while maintaining eye contact with a partner opposite you, as you sit alongside other pairings in rows. There are various White Tantric yoga events held all over the world (which can be found at www. whitetantricyoga.com). You can go along with a partner (it can be very beautiful and transformative to go along with an attachment figure, if they are willing) or you can go alone and partner-up while you are there.

Here are a few simple exercises from this tradition which you might like to try for yourself. However, when practised outside of a group, they do not constitute White Tantric yoga, as the diagonal energy is not present (White Tantra works on the movement of energy in zigzag lines down the rows of partners). However, these exercises can be a very good place to start to bring the sense of 'we' into the sense of 'I' and vice versa. Venus Kriyas from the Kundalini tradition are also a beautiful practice to this end.

When persuading a romantic partner or an attachment figure (e.g., your mother) to engage in these exercises with you, it might be useful to offer the following invitations and explanations:

- 'I have understood that some of my struggles might be connected to our relationship, particularly the relationship we had while I was growing up. I am not blaming you. I know that you did the very best you could, given your own experiences. I take my part of the responsibility for my struggles, too. I think it would be good to work through a few things together. What do you think?'

- 'I have come across these exercises that help people to connect more deeply. I'd really like to experience a deeper connection with you. Is this something you want also? If so, perhaps we could give this a try.'

- 'I know some of this might seem a bit weird or strange, but that's probably just because we are not used to doing things like this in our culture. People in other cultures engage in practices like this all the time. Have you seen or heard about tribes who work through their emotional pain by chanting, drumming, and dancing? I think this is rather like that.'

- 'Apparently, this might make us feel a bit uncomfortable at first or might make us giggle a bit. Let's just go with it anyway. What have we got to lose?'

- 'I have heard these practices can bring up a lot of emotional stuff. This might not be easy. Are you up for this? We can talk things through together afterwards if you like.'

- 'It would mean a lot to me if we could spend around eleven minutes (or whatever time frame you feel comfortable with) doing this together. You have been on my mind a lot, and our relationship is important to me. I think this could also really help me move on a bit, and perhaps also help you move on a bit, too. What do you think? Let's give it a whirl!'

Example Exercise One: Hummee Hum Brahm Hum with Palms Touching

The mantra 'Hummee Hum Brahm Hum' means, 'We are we and we are one'. There are some lovely recordings of this mantra you can use, such as those by Kevin James and Mirabai Ceiba. You can start with eleven minutes if you are new to this (you can set a timer to negate either of you having to be focused on the clock or you could use one of the recordings of a specific length). Sit opposite one another at eye-level, perhaps in easy-pose (with legs crossed) or rock pose (sitting on the heels). You can sit on chairs if injuries or discomfort are present. Hold up the palms of your hands at shoulder-height and connect with the palms of the person opposite you. Push gently into their palms as they, in turn, push gently into yours. Maintain this posture as you gaze into one another's eyes while singing along to the mantra, which is very easy to pick up.

Example Exercise Two: Hummee Hum Brahm Hum with Arms Extended

This version may be a little more physically challenging. You might like to try it after completing eleven minutes of the first exercise. Extend your right arm up at a diagonal (as though pointing to around two o'clock on a clock face), palm facing forwards. Connect with the left palm of your partner. At the same time, extend your left arm down at a diagonal (as though pointing to around eight o'clock on a clock face), connecting with your partner's right palm. Maintain a lengthened spine and extended arms as you repeat the period of chanting, 'Hummee Hum Brahm Hum,' while gazing into your partner's eyes.

Example Exercise Three: Hummee Hum Brahm Hum with Moving Arms

Extend your arms with a slight bend in the elbow, palms forward, interlacing your fingers with those of your partner's, both of your palms touching. Create a cycling motion with your arms, as though you are pedalling a bicycle with your partner's arms. Maintain a steady, even pace as you hold eye contact and repeat the period of chanting. It might be that you started with eleven minutes for the first two exercises, moving to thirty-one minutes for this dynamic exercise.

Follow-Up Conversations

We may find that engaging in exercises like these brings up a lot for us emotionally, psychologically, and spiritually. Taking time to be with the other person, whether this means sitting in silence, going for walk, or having a conversation together etc. is likely to create additional benefits. Conversely, it is also important to notice when enough has been said or shared presently and it is time to part ways and spend some time processing your experiences alone. You can always come back together later to talk, reconnect, or relationally engage in whichever way is desired/needed.

The following might be helpful pointers for follow-up discussions:

- 'How was that for you?'
- 'I am feeling [describe your feelings]. What feelings are coming up for you?'
- 'When I looked into your eyes, I felt [describe your feelings]. I think this might be because [describe why]. What do you think? How did you feel when you looked into my eyes?'
- 'I found that memories came up for me, like [describe your memories]. This made me feel [describe your feelings] and think of [describe your thoughts]. It makes me wonder about [describe your insights].'
- 'Did any memories come up for you?'
- 'The [name aspect of the experience] helped me feel things from your point of view, like [describe your insights]. I wonder if you might have felt [describe their feelings] when [describe a moment of importance]?'

- 'I felt a longing in myself for [describe your desires].'
- 'I found myself grieving for [describe your loss]. I wonder how we can move on together.'
- 'I am sorry for the times I [describe your regrets].'
- 'I wish we could have [describe past desires] when I was younger; although, I understand why things were the way they were.'
- 'I have learned a lot from being in relationship with you, like [describe your learnings].'
- 'I felt the presence of [name the person whose presence you felt while engaged in the exercise]. I think they came to mind because they [describe why]. What do you think? I wonder what they would say if they were here now.'
- 'I am grateful for this time with you.'
- 'I would like to hug you. Can I?'
- 'Would you like to go for a walk or have a cup of tea?'
- 'I feel like I need some space right now. Is it okay if I call you later or tomorrow?'

In secure attachment relationships, the cycle of 'rupture and repair' enables a continuing connection with the attachment figure. If this does not happen, there can be a sense of an ongoing, cavernous rupture, so large and all-encompassing that we can hardly imagine ever building bridges with the other person. Yet, it is never too late to begin taking small steps towards them; although, this always comes with a risk. What if they step away from us as we step towards them? What if they are not ready? What if they do not have the emotional capacity or it is too emotionally painful for them to find some semblance of repair with us? What if they reject us?

These are all possibilities. These possibilities can stop us from even attempting any repair, since the possible pain of rejection (all over again) feels too huge to bear. While it can be useful to ask ourselves if we feel emotionally strong enough to risk repeated rejection, it is also useful to remember that we are *always* emotionally strong enough, even if it does not feel like it. We have the capacity to bear any pain, no matter how vast. After all, have we not survived each of the painful emotional experiences of our lives up to this point (even if we have had to dissociate or escape into self-soothing behaviours in order to do so)?

It may be the case that our attachment figure simply doesn't want to go there in terms of repairing their relationship with us. This avoidance is also an invitation for our acceptance. It might also be that the body-mind of our attachment figure has died, and therefore, we feel like we no longer have the same opportunities for repair that we had when they were alive. Beautifully, a multitude of opportunities are still open to us, even if the body-minds of our attachment figures are no longer alive or do not want to engage in repair with us. The following meditation and the meditations/exercises offered in the next chapter (Chapter Nine) are just some such opportunities.

Meditation for Repairing Relationships 'Alone'

Call to mind the essence of your attachment figure as you sit quietly, alone. Close your eyes if this helps you focus and really feel into the sense of this person. Notice where the sense of them seems to sit within your body. How does your breathing pattern alter when you place your attention on the felt-sense of their personhood? Are there any changes in your posture? Where do your thoughts go?

Take long, deep breaths, using your breath to anchor yourself in the present moment and provide a sense of control and safety. If you feel afraid, feel into the fear also, inviting the felt-sense of your allies (other people, animals, or plants in your life who bring, or have brought, you comfort and a sense of safety).

Notice any visual images that arise in your awareness. Perhaps it is the person's face. Perhaps it is a visual memory of a time you spent with them. Notice any other senses that are activated also. Do you recall how the person smelled? The sound of their voice? Any tastes you associate with them? Any touch-sensations?

Stay with any thoughts, memories, sensations, or perceptions that arise. Take your stand as Love, witnessing these sensations emerging and dissolving without trying to escape from them or cling to them. Continue to use your breath as an anchor if this helps you.

Call this person's eyes into your mind and imagine gazing into them. Take your time with this. Alternatively, you might like to imagine holding their hand, sitting back-to-back with them (this can feel less threatening), walking along the beach with them, or wherever your inclinations take you.

Stay with any feelings that come up, as opposed to distracting yourself from them or pushing them away. Welcome these feelings like long-lost friends, with open arms and an open heart. If tears come, allow yourself to cry. Allow whatever is naturally flowing to flow without resisting any part of it. If thoughts and feelings of anger come, let them come. Feel into the anger fully, expressing it however it feels most spontaneous and natural to do so.

After you have taken some time to deeply feel any emotions without resistance, return to the sense/image person and do whatever feels natural to do in your mind's eye. This might be smiling at them, giving them a hug, patting their shoulder, offering them a flower, or something else entirely. There are no rights or wrongs. Simply go with your natural and spontaneous inclinations. You might find yourself feeling moved to express anger to them before you are able to express an act of forgiveness. Allow yourself to do or say whatever spontaneously emerges, however bombastic it might seem.

Whatever your experience has been, take time to thank this person and commend yourself for your bravery. You might like to write a letter to this person afterwards, expressing all that has taken place in your heart. You may like to keep this letter, or you may wish to put it in a bottle and throw it into the sea, burn it, read it to a trusted friend, respond to it as though you were the other person, and so on.

Regardless of whether the person is there in physicality or whether they are willing to engage with us, the most important element of our repair will be the feeling of our emotions attached to our relationship with them. Every avoidant behaviour we have ever engaged in—every binge, every skipped meal, every session of over-exercise, every self-criticism in front of the mirror—have all been (usually unconscious) attempts to avoid the emotions connected to painful relationships. Therefore, moving beyond our pain can be achieved by welcoming and fully experiencing our emotions. This is the work. This is the invitation. Within this act of courage lies the eventual lived experience of freedom.

Chapter Nine

Heal Your Current Relationships

Romantic relationships can be places where societal myths rear their heads very strongly. Just as our relationship with our bodies and food can mirror our early and/or current relationships with our primary caregivers, so, too, can our romantic relationships reflect the way we feed and treat our bodies. Thoughts may suggest that our romantic partner wants or even needs us to look a certain way for them to desire us and remain with us. Our romantic partner may even tell us this is the case, and thought could suggest that this is a legitimate reason for us to diet, have cosmetic surgery, and so on. So conditioned have we become that we may also make these demands of our partner. At the truest part of ourselves, our love is not attached to the size of our partner's belly; yet, we may find ourselves making wry comments about their weight or talking about their physical form in subtly derogatory ways.

More than this, our romantic relationships can become replicas of our primary attachment relationships if any unprocessed emotional pain remains. In this way, trauma connected to our primary caregiving relationships can continue to play itself out in our romantic relationships in a bid for resolution. We tend to repeat that which we do not repair. Emotional debris will utilise any opportunity and non-opportunity to be felt and assimilated. Alongside this, we tend to keep our patterns and to repeat them because if they are relinquished we will create a black hole, a vacuum. Something in our body-mind nature abhors a vacuum so we would rather repeat destructive patterns than create silence, emptiness and spaciousness.

My relationship with my husband is an example of this. My early relationship with my mother was insecure. I felt I had to hide away my natural beingness and organic inclinations to be acceptable to her, in order not to frighten her away. To remain connected to my mother, it was necessary to abandon my emotions and my spontaneity to a certain extent. Over time, I increasingly became a wooden puppet, an emotionless being whose sole aim was to be the 'good girl' I unconsciously understood I needed to be.

Of course, my mother yearned for me to be 'perfect' because she herself had experienced considerable attachment-based trauma in her own childhood, alongside numerous other traumas. Thus, history began to repeat itself, as it so often does.

When I met my husband, I had not yet worked through my attachment-based pain. I didn't really even know it was there yet.

It was very complicated between myself and my husband in the early years of our relationship for all sorts of reasons. Regardless, I jumped into our liaison with both feet. It is not unusual for people who have experienced insecure early caregiver attachment patterns to do this. I wanted to kiss him right away, move in with him straight away, and marry him tomorrow! Understandably, this seemed to scare him off a bit. As it was, my husband wanted to take things very slowly. A wise person once said that in every romantic relationship there is one person who fears being abandoned and one person who fears losing themselves. It was clear which of each myself and my husband were very early on. It took a fair few years for us to move in together, get married, and many other aspects besides.

The waiting was experienced as painful by my body-mind. Why didn't my boyfriend want me? Why didn't he wish to live with me and marry me? All the old feelings of not being good enough rose to the surface, alongside my core belief that I was a person who was difficult to love.

I cried a lot in those years. My later-to-be-husband was doing the best he could do, and it would not have been right for him to concede moving forward in our relationship before he was ready. Yet, I ached for concrete 'proof' that I was loved and accepted by him. At times, he would move in with me for a couple of weeks and then move back out again. Later, he would live and work abroad for over three years. Some of his expressive behaviours, in many ways, became the perfect mirror for the push-pull relationship I had with my mother growing up—*I want you; I do not want you as you are. You are good enough; you are not good enough.*

When I allowed myself to admit it, I knew I was absolutely terrified of being abandoned by my husband. Each of my husband's actions that seemed to be ambivalent or avoidant were viscerally frightening for me.

In the yogic tradition, it is believed that body-minds choose their parents. At 120 days after conception, a soul chooses to incarnate through the womb of a woman. This notion blows the reasoning of blaming our mother for our experiences clean out of the water. On a deeper level, we chose the experiences we would have in this body in order to further evolve on this journey to the heart. Whether or not your beliefs align with this notion, you can perhaps agree that most of us choose our romantic partners. Part of my attraction to my husband was his similarity to my mother. I did not notice this until many years into our relationship. It was unconscious and implicit in so many ways.

Of course, there were many other reasons I was attracted to my husband. The most fundamental of these reasons is that this was to be our path—that we would marry and journey along together. As with everything else in life, it could not have been any other way.

My husband is a wonderful human being. He is also a human being who has brought my emotional pain to the surface in the strongest of ways (as have I, for him, in turn). The two are not mutually exclusive. I am deeply grateful to my husband for the pain our relationship has thrown up over the years.

The emotional pain in our lives is always a portal into growth, healing, and remembering who we truly are.

At certain points in my life, my relationship with my mother was based on fear. My relationship with food and my body was based on fear. My relationship with my husband was based on fear—fear of him abandoning me and fear that I was not worthy of his love.

These three relationships—with my mother, with food/my body, and with my husband—were totally tangled up. I would try to address one of these relationships and then find myself struggling with another. I was passing the buck between my mother, my husband, and food continuously. At least one part of the triad received my fearful focus at any one time. I was continually trying to 'fix' one of these aspects in whichever way I could, or indeed, attempting to avoid the emotional pain related to one of these relationships during any given period.

At some point, I realised the very same fear was underlying my suffering within each of these three relationships. The fear of my perceived unlovability underpinned them all.

I had two options, as I then saw it. I could continue to struggle with my husband, my mother, and food, or I could place my awareness on the underlying pain and fear. At some point, I realised life would continue to find new and innovative ways of dredging up my core sense of unlovability until I dived into it, heard the story it was trying to tell me and assimilated it into my wholeness.

At a certain point, I understood that the pain related to my relationship with my husband was inviting me to acknowledge and feel my early attachment-based pain. However, I continued to cry inconsolably each time my husband flew off to Germany and continued to experience pain in the pit of my stomach when he told me he would be staying away for another stretch of time. I noticed a difference between the tears that came because I missed my husband, which were a quiet sort of tears without any self-pity embedded in them, to the kind of tears I felt totally torn apart by. The former kind of tears were the simple expression of the deep connection I had with my husband. The latter were an expression of my early attachment history. Both needed to be felt, but to ascribe the latter tears to my husband was not serving our relationship. These tears were begging to be returned to the place where they belonged—to my sense of unlovability, rooted in my developmental history. When I welcomed my core sense of unlovability and allowed myself to truly feel it, my relationship with my husband blossomed in the most beautiful and profound way.

Yogi Bhajan explained that emotion can either become commotion or devotion. In the early years of our relationship, my emotion often turned to commotion in relation to my husband. I regularly found my unresolved emotional pain being 'triggered' by him. I would then leap into blaming the absence of my husband for my upset. Of course, we are never upset for the reasons we think we are. My husband was not to blame for my sadness or tears. They were not his responsibility, nor could they have ever been. As my relationship with my husband has deepened and developed over the past decade, I have come to recognise the following pointers as incredibly helpful in terms of transmuting emotion into devotion, as opposed to commotion:

- Remember that the other person is you (this is one of Yogi Bhajan's mantras for the Aquarian Age).
- Always assume the other person has good intentions.
- Do not make any other assumptions.
- Throw out all expectations. Meet the person as though you are encountering them for the very first time.
- Check things out before drawing any conclusions: 'When you said x, I felt y. Is this what you meant/intended?'
- When triggered, look into the person's eyes. Touch them with one hand if they allow you to, bringing your other

hand to your heart. Connect with your heart centre and relate to your partner from this place (not from the intellect). Breathe deeply. Immerse your awareness in the love you feel for this person. Recall a time when you felt completely at One with them, and they felt completely at One with you.

- Thank the person for bringing your unresolved emotional stuff to the surface. Now, it can be heard and healed.

Reassurance-seeking is an example of emotion becoming commotion, epitomised by the proverbial phrase, *'Does my bum look big in this?'* When we enter a cycle of reassurance-seeking with our romantic partner, we set both of us up to fail. Notice that your partner's answer to your reassurance-seeking, whatever it might be, can never truly satisfy you. Notice also that such reassurance-seeking puts your relationship very securely on the superficial level of body-mind relating to body-mind. You did not meet your partner to relate to them on a body-mind to body-mind level. You met them to experience dissolution of the subject and object. You met them to advance on your spiritual journey and your quest to return to your true Self. You met them to experience the Love you intrinsically are.

When we seek reassurance about our appearance, we are seeking security and connection. We want to feel safe. We yearn to collapse the seeking energy to feel secure. It is far more effective to bypass the smokescreen and go directly to the source of our desire. We can do this by candidly seeking a connection to our partner, such as by initiating a hug, reaching out to hold their hand, taking some silent moments to gaze into their eyes, and so on. When the urge to seek reassurance from our partner arises, we can respond to this urge by making a heart-to-heart connection. Then, the need to chase after a sense of security and safety will melt away.

The following responses can be helpful when our partner

seeks appearance-focused reassurance from us. You might like to share these example responses with your partner if you are the one who tends to engage in the reassurance-seeking:

- 'I can sense that you are feeling a bit unsafe right now. Would it help to have a hug, to spend some time meditating together, or to go for a walk while holding hands?'
- 'I am more interested in what you plan to do in that pair of jeans than what you look like in them.'
- 'It appears you are seeking reassurance from me. I want to reassure you that I see you, I hear you, and I love you.'
- 'I want to remind you that you are not your body. You are the one who is aware of your body. You are a spirit having a human experience. You are Love. I am that same Love. We are One.'

Sex can become a minefield when we feel insecure about the appearance of our body. The idea of 'getting naked' and being touched can be terrifying (particularly if we have experienced any form of sexual abuse—which has a much higher rate in the disordered eating population than the general population). We may be afraid that we will put our partners off, repulse them, or even scare them away. It can be incredibly helpful to be open to our partner about our fears. We might like to say something like, *'I feel really insecure about my belly. I feel like it is too big and wobbly. I am afraid you will be disgusted if you see and touch it. I feel ashamed. I want to feel comfortable with you seeing and touching my belly but the sheer idea of it fills me with dread.'* Having shared our truth, it will be important for us to spend time feeling into the sensations and emotions connected to our impressions of our belly. We can do this alone or alongside our partner, perhaps by asking them to gently place their hand on our belly as we feel into any sensations and emotions that arise. It can be beautiful and beneficial to try out some of the following:

- Spend time exploring your partner's body, perhaps with some mantras playing and some incense or candles burning. Spend time exploring the part of your partner's body which you have a hard time with in relation to your own body. For example, if you dislike your legs, spend extra time exploring your partner's legs. Welcome any emotions that emerge as a result. Invite your partner to do the same with your body, particularly directing them towards your feared parts. It can be very powerful to say 'hello' to each part of the body as you and your partner explore them. For example, try saying, 'Hello, belly,' while offering your partner's belly a tender kiss.
- Invite your partner to photograph, paint, draw, and/or sculpt your feared body part.
- Invite your partner to slowly and tenderly touch, kiss, massage, and embrace your feared body part.
- Invite your partner to draw or paint love hearts, personal symbols or whatever else they feel moved to draw or paint on your feared body part. Little essential oil rollers can be a lovely way to do this.
- Connect body-part to body-part with your partner. For example, press your belly against theirs, entangle your legs with theirs, or connect chest-to-chest with them. Breathe deeply as you begin to lose the sense of where your body part ends and their body part begins.

In so much as we recognise that the other person is us, we also recognise that our body is their body and their body is our own. There is no separation. As we fall in love with our partner's arms, so, too, can we fall in love with *our* arms. Sex can be a beautiful expression of this Oneness, this timeless union. Yet, we do not need to have full, penetrative sex to experience this (though, at times, we might choose to experience it in this way). We can experience this Oneness with a simple look, a heartfelt touch, or a sincere word. There have been many occasions when I have caught the gaze of my husband and felt any sense of separation between us melt effortlessly. In these moments, there is no my-body and his-body. There is simply This. Simply Aliveness expressing itself. Simply Love.

We can also feel the emotions related to past attachment relationships through current attachment relationships, and then we can work through them. The issue is not that we often tend to work through historic attachment-based pain in current attachment relationships but that we *often do not realise this is what we are doing.* When we notice patterns of behaviour in current relationships that hark back to earlier attachment relationships, we can begin to actively engage in the healing process, as opposed to being swept unconsciously into vicious cycles. The vicious cycles can, thus, become virtuous cycles. The following exercise might support you in this.

Exploring and Releasing Historic Attachment-Based Pain in Current Relationships

Note any areas of your current relationship (this might be a romantic relationship or another close relationship) which you prefer were different in some way. For example, you might wish that your partner listened to your point of view more often, that they (or you) could be less jealous, or that you could spend less time in conflict... whatever it might be.

Write down any core-thoughts that tend to come up linked to each of these areas. For example, if you wish your partner listened to your point of view more closely, linked thoughts might be: 'He doesn't care about me'; 'He doesn't find me interesting'; 'He's too wrapped up in himself to notice me.' Allow some of the pushed-away, catastrophic thoughts to come up and write them down also. For example: 'He doesn't love me'; 'He doesn't care a toss for me'; 'He thinks everyone is more interesting than I am'; 'I am a boring person'; 'I am not worth listening to'; 'I disgust him'; 'He will leave me eventually.'

Now, take some time to write down any linked emotions. Try to get to the core emotion if you can, which will ultimately be rooted in the fear of being unlovable. Types of associated emotions that might come up could be abandonment, shame, guilt, unworthiness, anger, jealousy, and grief.

Take some time to feel into the core emotions you have written down. Invite the emotions in, noticing where they are felt in your body. Fully feel into any associated sensations that emerge.

Allow any memories to come to the surface. Allow resistance to surface without acting on it. Do not resist the resistance. The memories that emerge might be explicit memories or implicit memories, meaning they may reveal themselves through thoughts or through your bodily sensations and impressions, or maybe both.

Feel into any links between these core emotions and your early attachment relationships. Notice how you have been trying to avoid these emotions to protect yourself from the painful experiences and memories of your attachment history. This has been an adaptive response and is absolutely nothing to berate yourself for. All human beings do this to varying degrees and this avoidance will have surely served you at some point in the past. Welcome the recognition that this avoidance is no longer serving you.

Imagine yourself as a tiny infant, totally helpless, unable to defend yourself and unable to make sense of your painful experiences. Again, feel into any associated emotional pain without resistance. If you could have responded or fought back as an infant, what would you have done? See yourself doing this in your mind's eye. What would you have said? Say it, either in the silence of your heart or out loud.

Bring the face of your current attachment figure (i.e., your romantic partner) into your mind's eye. Acknowledge that you have been playing out some of your early attachment history with this person in addition to projecting undigested relational experiences on to them. Thank them for being the receptacle of some of your pain. If you feel able, make a commitment to them to notice when you are triggered, and to be honest with yourself and them about these triggers as they arise. Acknowledge *that you may not always notice and may continue to play old patterns out in a bid to resolve them. Tell the other person how they can help you with this, for example: Gently pointing out when your reaction appears to be disproportionate to the event; supporting you emotionally when you are triggered by hugging you and listening without trying to 'fix' anything; and being open and honest with you in turn when their own historical attachment-based pain is triggered.*

This might all take place entirely in your imagination or you might like to have a conversation with your partner, which can be incredibly helpful. You might say something like, 'I have noticed that I tend to get really angry with you when you don't tell me what time you are coming home. I know this has been quite a source of conflict for us. I am sorry. I have recently come to realise that I may get so upset about this because I was so often left alone as an infant. I never knew if or when my mother would be coming when I wanted her, and this probably terrified me. I probably felt as though I was going to die, because I was unable to meet my own needs, such as feeding myself and keeping myself warm. I probably subconsciously deduced that I was unlovable. Now, I react as though I am going to die—as though it is the end of the world—when I feel uncertain about what time you are coming home. I know this sounds extreme but I believe this is how it is. I also probably unconsciously assume that your desire to be out is an indicator that you do not love me.

I would really appreciate your patience with me. It would help if you could tell me, whenever it is possible, approximately what time you are coming home. I know this isn't always possible, though. At those times, I will try to remember that I seem to get so upset about this because I haven't fully processed the terror I experienced as an infant when I didn't know when my mother would return and/or if I deserved her attention and love. If I forget, I wouldn't mind you reminding me, although I may not always thank you for it at the time if my panic is very high. I could also do with a hug/kiss/squeeze of the shoulder etc. when you come home. It really helps me calm down when I feel physically close to you.'

Chapter Ten

Fall into the Metaphor

Appearance-focused identity struggles are always rooted in the fear of being unlovable and, therefore, in a lack of self-love. They are literally a metaphor for a lack of self-love. For this reason, they regularly go together with other practices and metaphors that express a lack of love and acceptance of the self. These might include compulsions, self-harm (now often referred to as 'self-injurious behaviour' in clinical literature), and engaging in undermining romantic relationships, to name but a few.

The compulsive seeking of cosmetic, dermatological, and dental procedures is not uncommon for people who pin their identities on to their physical appearance. It is especially common for people with a diagnosis of BDD. There is often a sense that once a perceived defect in the physical appearance is 'fixed', the person will feel lovable and all shall be well. This is not borne out in my personal and clinical experience, nor in my research into BDD. Rather, once one 'appearance-project' has been completed, the person tends to move their focus to another aspect of their appearance. This makes complete sense when we consider that these struggles are never about the appearance at their core, but rather are rooted in low self-esteem, lack of self-worth, and flailing self-acceptance and self-love.

There are two seemingly opposing arguments for practices like cosmetic surgery. These could be seen, to borrow terms from Robert Brian, the author of *The Decorated Body*, as the 'figuration' argument and the 'disfiguration' argument. The 'figuration' argument suggests that practices like cosmetic surgery can be self-affirming. Some people talk about their surgeries as helping them to 'become who they always felt they were', for example. The 'disfiguration' argument, on the other side of the coin, views these practices as self-destructive. The cosmetic surgery, or whatever else it may be, is sought out, unconsciously, as a self-destructive act and serves only to take the person further away from the remembering and experience of their true Self. It would certainly appear to be the case that those seeking cosmetic surgery and similar practices to somehow 'fix' their appearance or to increase their self-esteem and perceived lovability are rarely (if ever) satisfied with the outcome. Rather, their attention typically moves to another aspect of their appearance, as the underlying sense of being 'not good enough' and unlovable remains.

As we have explored, the practices we seek out to amend our bodies are typically metaphors for our early caregiving relationships, given that our sense of our body emerges within the context of these early relationships. Of course, it is through the primary caregiver that the infant organises its early bodily sensations and experiences; thus, coming to its sense of a body-self. The experience of touch is central to this. Not only the regularity of touch but also, and very importantly, the quality and tenderness of touch. An infant who is held awkwardly will sense the awkwardness and amend its behaviour to obtain more certain, secure physical contact.

The seeing of the infant by the caregiver is an implicit element of contact comfort, so much so that psychologist and psychoanalyst Alessandra Lemma refers to it as the 'gaze-touch relationship'. Touch and gaze would appear to be inseparable within the early infant experience. Perhaps they remain inseparable throughout our lives. Lemma suggests that when there are difficulties within the early touch-gaze relationship with the primary caregiver(s), it can prove impossible to feel at home in one's body, or even to feel that one 'has' a body; that the body is one's own. She goes on to suggest that during adolescence difficulties can arise when the body presents itself strongly to the mind, partially because of the many changes it undergoes. It may then follow that the body is 'blamed' for the inner pain and turmoil experienced by the person in thought and sensation. This can make it even more difficult to assimilate the body into the sense of who the person is. Since the body is deemed to be at 'fault' for the sense of a fragmented self, the body is felt to need changing or 'fixing' to reduce or abolish any emotional pain. In many cases, the body is blamed for the felt sense of unlovability, often leading to the belief that once the body is changed or 'fixed', the person will become lovable and 'whole'.

Sigmund Freud, Donald Winnicott, and others have argued that the body-self is the foundation of the sense of self. Therefore, for change in the conceptualisation of the self to take place, one must necessarily arrive at a sense of the body-self. We cannot divorce the body from our experience. Neither can we expect our sense of self to be altered, in any lasting way, by amending the appearance of the body. The relationship of the self to the body is not appearance-related but, rather, related to the early development of the self, which happened through the body.

It is possible for a split to occur between the body-mind. The mind can be conceived of and experienced as the self, while the body is experienced and conceived of as the 'other'. It is this 'othering' that enables the belief that the self can amend the body, and that it is possible to exert control over the body; in other words, 'me' as a mind, changing the 'body' in order to become a whole 'me' or a better version of 'me'. Perhaps there is a notion that once the body is altered to look the way thought suggests it should look, this body can then, and *only* then, be fully assimilated into the lived sense of self. It is, of sorts, a kind of splitting—the current body as 'all bad' and the thoughts of changing it as 'all good'. The hope, perhaps, is to transmute the body into the 'good object' in order to create a cohesive, 'good self'—or, at least, the outward appearance of a 'good self'—to ensure desirability and, therefore, the experience of being loved.

Just as our rejection of food can play out our early felt

rejection by our primary caregiver, so, too, can our desire to amend the body live out this rejection. Our rejection of our physical appearance mirrors our unconscious rejection of either separation from, or enmeshment with, the caregiver. The 'other' who is the caregiver is replaced with the 'other' of the idealised body. The person becomes infatuated with the image of their body as thinner, less blemished, more muscular etc., having what could be described as a relationship between their current self (their current mirror image) and their projected, idealised self (their idealised, desired future mirror image). This relationship replaces the enmeshed relationship with the caregiver. It is a desperate bid to separate from this enmeshment.

As we aim to transmute the physical appearance into something 'beautiful' and 'lovable', so, too, do we unconsciously strive to transmute our early relationship, and all it stood for, into something beautiful and good. We attempt to make sense of our early and most important relationships through the body. How and where else, after all, could we make sense of them, given that it is through the body that these early relationships emerge?

The experience of shame would appear to underscore the primary reasons that most us attempt to amend the physical appearance of our body. This experience of shame is also fundamentally rooted in the body-self. If we did not often have the experience of being 'good enough' as infants, an overwhelming sense of shame can take an insidious anchor in our body-experience. This shame often sits between the experiences of not being 'desirable' as a human being and being 'swallowed up' as an individual self by another, usually a primary caregiver.

Shame lodged in the body negates the possibility to feel safe in the body. People whose bodies are permeated by shame typically have a sense of a fragmented body or an inability to experience a lived sense of the body. They use metaphors like 'being in pieces', 'feeling disconnected', or 'feeling dead from the neck down'. These inner impressions regularly play themselves out through a person's dreams and nightmares, such as in the form of dreams of objects being embedded in or emerging from the flesh, dreams of being unable to feel parts of the body, and dreams of parts of the body going missing or becoming maimed or dismembered. Regularly, the dreams take on an observer perspective in which the dreamer is nobody in the dream and is rather a floating 'nothingness' passively observing all that comes to pass. Sometimes, the felt sense of being nobody and having no body is projected on to another figure in the dream. Perhaps this 'other' is transparent or translucent. Perhaps they have missing limbs. Perhaps their body 'falls apart', 'withers away', or takes on a grotesque form.

The sense of shame living within the body is a difficult one to describe. Oftentimes, it emerges as a sense that we don't fit our bodies somehow. Or it might feel like we do not belong 'in the body' or we perceive ourselves as an imposter within our body. We do not feel 'at home' in our body, and rather, we experience perhaps a sense of entrapment or misalignment. We can try to make sense of this in a myriad of ways and it is not uncommon to look towards society to inform and direct our thinking. If we are living in a society that suggests we can feel better about ourselves by altering the appearance of our body, as indeed many of us are, then it makes sense that we might take this on as an identity project.

It is through the body, in early infancy, that we come to a lived sense of our corporeality. If our early experiences have been esteeming, we are likely to develop a sense of comfort and safety as/within a physical body. If, on the other hand, our early experiences have been undermining, a sense of being a 'bad body' is more likely to emerge.

If the 'desiring' gaze of the other is absent in infancy, Lemma conjectures it often follows that the person will later search for the loving gaze in whichever mirrors are available. These mirrors could be other people or reflective surfaces such as actual mirrors. Rather than finding the loving gaze they are seeking, people whose infantile experiences were rooted in shame are likely to find 'more of the same'. This is partially due to a confirmation-bias within the psyche and partially because we tend to seek out relationships which will facilitate a resolution of early, unresolved experiences.

It is no secret that we often seek romantic partners who bear some level of physical, emotional, and/or psychological similarity to our primary caregiver(s) as we explored a little in the previous chapter. In them, do we perhaps unconsciously hope to soothe, make sense of, and transfigure our early attachment relationships. In them, do we perhaps unconsciously ache to see the desiring gaze we experienced as absent in our infancy. Through our liaison with them, do we perhaps unconsciously hope to gather the scattered fragments of ourselves, join with their fragments, and, thus, have an experience of being or becoming whole. We hope for the opportunity to be seen, touched, and loved, as well as to see, touch, and love in return.

My husband specialises in working with people who hear voices. As I began to open up to my husband about my self-loathing experiences pinned on to my physical appearance, we started, together, to draw parallels between myself and the people my husband supported. I believe these parallels can be drawn between people manifesting emotional struggles in all forms, since their root is ultimately the same. We might profess that we are nothing like people who hear voices. As such, we are utterly fooling ourselves. We are *absolutely* like people who hear voices, abuse alcohol, take illegal substances, and starve themselves. All body-minds are running away from something. And the Awareness that each of us are is the same Freedom. The same Aliveness. The same Love.

People who hear voices often experience these voices as being massively persecutory. They are often afraid of them and sometimes experience being 'driven mad' by them. Consequently, their wish is often to get rid of these voices, to be free of them, and to relinquish them in order to be able to move forward in their lives.

In his work with people who hear voices, my husband has found that the invitation is not to get rid of the voices but to welcome them and to listen openly to all that they are trying to express. When the emotional story the voices are trying to communicate has been heard, the voices then tend to disappear or assimilate of their own accord.

Human beings need metaphors. Direct verbalisations tend to be caught by thought, which then colours the meaning with heavy conditioning. Metaphors—such as in the form of poetry, works of art, and so on can initially bypass thought and, thus, strike to the centre of the soul. They can sidestep conditioning. Thus, we can stand in front of a painting or read a poem and find tears rolling unannounced down our unsuspecting cheeks. Somehow, the poem, the sculpture, the piece of music, or whatever else it might be, has expressed a part of our experience that slips between cognition and strikes to the very heart of truth. Metaphors glide past thought and make a direct beeline for the deepest knowing. This is why spiritual teachers throughout the ages have relied so heavily on metaphorical stories through which to communicate central truths and mystical knowings.

The voices people tend to hear usually speak in metaphors. They might say things like, *you should kill yourself* or *you need to set fire to your mother's house*. Sometimes, people take these invitations literally. Yet, the voices are expressing something else entirely.

When the person truly listens to their voices—ideally, without any attempt to push them away or get rid of them—they tend to arrive at a different understanding. They begin to hear metaphors. *You should kill yourself* becomes *your old life wants to die*, and *you need to set fire to your mother's house* becomes *your *freedom lies in walking away from your enmeshment with your mother.*

In the very same way, the 'voice' (which may have the sound of our own voice 'inside' our 'head') which implores us to lose weight, for example, is speaking in metaphors. The voice or thought that says, *you need to lose five pounds in order to be a good person*, is metaphorically imploring, *you need to drop something in order to remember that you already are a good person.*

Understanding a metaphor is a creative endeavour. Within metaphors, words take on new, extended meanings. Implicit in metaphor, then, is ambiguity. The 'aha' moment when the ambiguity is lifted and the meaning is revealed appears to take place beyond thought, perhaps in the space between thoughts. Thus, metaphor is used by the 'voices' as an outside-of-thought invitation.

The issue is not our voices or our thoughts but the fact that we have ascribed truth to them. We have decided that a thought which suggests that we need to lose five pounds in order to be lovable means we literally need to lose five pounds to become lovable. Outside of thought, the idea that the loss of five pounds would make anything or anyone lovable is preposterous. The five pounds are a metaphor for all that we need to lose, all that is covering up the remembering of our intrinsic lovability. Society suggests that losing weight will make us more lovable, so thought uses that. But between the thoughts in the 'aha' moment of the metaphor, it is understood that our sole desire (and, indeed, our soul's desire) is only ever to remember who we truly are.

Appearance-focused suffering always comes back to the core belief of the body-mind that the body-mind self is bad. *Too fat* is, itself, a metaphor for *bad*. *Bad* is a metaphor for, *you have forgotten who you truly are. You have forgotten that you are Love.*

Metaphors demand not that we look at the concrete words or manifestations but that we allow ourselves to freefall into the space between the words or images. The invitation is implicit, as the memory and experience are, themselves, implicit. We rarely hold concrete, explicit memories for our developmental traumas. They are typically just beyond the grasp of our cognition. In the same way, the concrete words and behaviours of our metaphors gently shield the semi-translucent truth of our experiences. It is within this truth that our freedom is to be rediscovered.

It doesn't help that the medical model often prefers to focus on concrete words and behaviours. The predominant medical model for supporting people who experience emotional distress is either to medicate them or talk to them (i.e., 'talking therapies'). For example, treatment for anorexia typically involves behaviour modification through meal plans, a reduction of exercise, and weigh-ins, alongside talking therapy, perhaps with a dose of antidepressants and/or anti-anxiety medication thrown in. Similarly, the predominant treatment for body dysmorphic disorder is Cognitive Behavioural Therapy (CBT) with Exposure and Response Prevention (ERP), with its focus being on amending thoughts, feelings, and behaviours, alongside high doses of selective serotonin reuptake inhibitors (SSRIs). While I am not disavowing the potential benefits of approaches such as these, which can prove hugely beneficial to a great many people, I am concerned that they often seem to miss the implicit, procedural 'talk' of the body and neglect the metaphor behind that which can be seen and heard.

The following case study of Julia serves to illustrate this point.

Julia received a diagnosis of body dysmorphic disorder following two years of agonising over the shape of her nose. Julia had spent up to three hours a day for the past two years in front of the mirror, inspecting her nose from every angle and shedding many tears over what she considered to be its asymmetry and large size. Julia also spent multiple hours a day on the Internet looking for cosmetic procedures to 'fix' her nose, in addition to spending hundreds of pounds on concealers to make her nose appear smaller. Julia had given up her job in design eight months previously, as it had become too difficult for her to get herself ready in time each morning due to her long ritual of applying cosmetics. Julia found it incredibly painful to leave the house and face the world with what she considered to be her 'hideous defect'.

Julia's psychological treatment largely focused on reducing her safety behaviours (such as checking her nose in the mirror and other reflective surfaces, reapplying cosmetics throughout the day, avoiding certain lighting, and speaking to people only from a certain angle), and exposing herself to the activities of daily living she had been avoiding. This helped a great deal, and Julia was increasingly able to engage in social activities and was beginning to think about returning to work. However, she noticed that she was now becoming preoccupied with other aspects of her appearance, such as the thinning of her hair and the facial skin around her jawline. Julia tried to apply the techniques she had learned in treatment to these emerging concerns but felt unable to keep up with how fast her body dysmorphia seemed to move and how rapidly it found new ways of seemingly torturing her.

Julia continued to work concertedly on amending her behaviours to stay on top of her BDD. Some days, she felt able to keep her head above water, and other days, she felt herself sinking beneath the surface — 'not waving but drowning'. Exhausted, Julia began to wonder about her focus on her nose, hair, and skin. When had this started? Why had she come to perceive defects in her physical appearance and why were they so distressing for her?

A range of difficult emotions came up when Julia asked herself these questions. This made her want to run in the opposite direction and to return her attention to her perceived 'too-big' nose, thinning hair, and blemished skin. Each time Julia asked herself these 'why' questions, she found herself returning to the mirror to inspect her appearance or touching her jawline to check for blemishes. Perhaps I am on to something here, she thought. Why do I return to my appearance when my emotions feel too big for me to handle? What would happen if I allowed myself to feel these emotions, as opposed to escaping them by staring into the mirror for hours?

Although she felt very frightened, Julia began to stay with the emotions attached to her perceived defects. She found that her perceived 'too-big' nose and other perceived appearance defects were her go-to-focus when feelings of shame came up. The sense of 'my nose is too big' was a metaphor for her shame, which was embedded in early-life experiences that had become implicitly stored in her body—initially, in her nose, in particular.

Julia considered how the nose is the organ of smell, which plays a key role in the bonding process in infancy. She noticed how it is the part of the face that protrudes more than any other, mapping to how painful she found it as a child to 'protrude' in her primary caregiver's awareness, as this usually resulted in admonishment and subsequent shame. Julia mused upon how the nose strongly relates to the sense of taste and how food was tangled up with a lack of connection in her early caregiving relationship. She also remembered how often her sister was praised for her 'cute button nose' when they were growing up and how such a nose became synonymous in her mind with nurture, since her sister always seemed to be much closer to her mother than herself.

Julia's hours of mirror gazing seemed to be a metaphor for Julia's search for her true Self. Julia had been looking for her true Self her whole life, having assumed a false self to more readily meet the needs and demands of her primary caregivers in infancy and while growing up. Her attempts to conceal the size of her nose by using carefully-researched-and-applied cosmetics was a metaphor for her need to hide in order to feel safe. In many ways, Julia was living in a painful dichotomy; wanting to be seen for who she truly was while feeling the need to hide who she was to avoid being shamed and rejected.

Julia's attempts to 'fix' her nose only served to heighten her focus on her nose and cause increasing shame. Often, the heavy layers of cosmetics she used on and around her nose **did** cause people's attention to be drawn to her nose, whereas they would not, ordinarily, have even noticed it. In the same way, some of Julia's safety behaviours, such as angling her body away from people as she spoke to them, ignited exactly the kind of perplexed looks she had been trying to avoid.

Julia started to put aside twenty minutes each morning to sit with *the sensations of her nose. She allowed any emerging sensations and emotions to be there, exactly as they were, without judging them or trying to escape from them. Many memories of different kinds came up and she cried many tears. Over time, Julia noticed that she no longer felt the compulsion to check her nose in the mirror, or indeed other aspects of her appearance. Her use of concealer and the compulsive touching of her skin seemed to fall away organically. Having felt the emotions connected to the experiences her nose and other aspects of her appearance were speaking to, she no longer had anything to avoid or to hate herself for. Julia understood that her desire to have a smaller nose and clearer skin were metaphors for her desire to be loved.*

When we fall into the metaphor behind our compulsions, we are regularly afforded a deep understanding of what our desires to amend our physical appearance are rooted in.

There are different parts, different aspects of ourselves that hold distinct information, experiences, and patterns. As children, these parts often felt a lot more tangible to us, perhaps in the form of imaginary friends, toys, character roles we took on in our play, and so on. As adults, we can lose touch with these parts and, therefore, with the experiences and memories they hold. To feel integrated and whole, it is important not to cut off, deny, or banish these aspects of ourselves. This includes those aspects of ourselves—those metaphors—related to our appearance-focused identity struggles. If I deny Ugliness as a part of myself, for example, I neglect the information and experiences that Ugliness speaks to and holds.

It can be helpful to interview the parts of ourselves we have been trying to 'fix', get rid of, or disconnect ourselves from. Below is an example of an interview I had with my sense of ugliness, which I had been trying to 'fix' by losing weight and clearing up my skin for many years. When we interview these rejected parts of ourselves, it is important to pose questions which hold in mind that the intention of these rejected parts is always good.

The invitation is to speak to these parts as though they came into our lives for a specific purpose and are benevolent in nature. We are invited to be open to their responses, whatever they may be.

We can either pose these questions to ourselves in the silence of our minds or aloud. Or we can hand the questions over to a trusted loved one or aligned professional to interview our rejected parts with and for us.

Interview with Ugliness

Ugliness, when did you first come into my life?

I came into your life before you were born, Nicole. Your parents had experienced a lot of attachment-based trauma, in addition to other traumas growing up. They were very young when they had you. Your mother was extremely anxious and stressed out while you were in the womb and you felt this. Then, when you were born, there was no space for your emotions or natural inclinations. Your mother was doing her best given her emotion resources; yet, you had to be the 'perfect' baby so that you would not frighten her away. It is impossible to be the perfect baby! So, you felt terrified much of the time. I stayed quiet at this point—my time had not yet come. But I was there from the very beginning.

So, when did you overtly come into my life in the form of Ugliness?

You might be surprised by this answer, but you were about three years old. You had already noticed at this point that you needed to look perfect, as well as behave perfectly. You noticed how upset your mother became if your hair was untidy, if you had food on your face, or if your clothing was creased or dirty. You had already figured out that 'looking pretty' was a way to please your mother and keep her close to you.

What would have happened if you had not come into my life?

If I had not come into your life, you would have continued to believe there was nothing you could do to become lovable. I gave you a project you could cling to. You focused on keeping your hair tidy, your clothes clean, and your skin clear, as well as maintaining a low weight. This gave you a sense that you were working towards a time when your mother would be pleased with you; thus, your true Self would be accepted and loved by her. This gave you hope. I gave you hope.

What would my mother say about why you came into my life?

She would say that I came into your life to punish her. She is right, in a way. Refusing food was the first and only time you went against your mother's expressed wishes. You needed to find a way to go against her desires to separate from her. I facilitated your retaliation against the unrealistic demands your mother was placing on you. I gave you a means to separate from your mother.

Are there other parts of me who are your friends or allies?

Yes. All the parts of yourself that make a bid for your freedom are my allies. Your courage, willingness to take risks, creativity, integrity, authenticity, and assertiveness are all my friends. By the same token, your gentleness, kindness, and compassion for yourself and others are my allies, too.

What is your purpose? What are you trying to achieve?

I am trying to bring you back to a sense that you are intrinsically lovable, just as you are. As you enter into the heart of the felt sense of me, you find that your beauty lies amidst the darkness, not outside of it.

I call you Ugliness. Is there another name you would like to be called, or which would be more fitting for you?

Stop pushing me away. Feel into me without judgement. Cry your tears for having been treated as though you are unlovable. Feel into this sense of unlovability. Then you will discover that my name is Freedom.

Chapter Eleven

Let Go of Compulsions

Just as our eating behaviours can say something about our early attachment relationships, so, too, can the methods we 'choose' to use to self-harm. Cutting of the skin is a metaphorical severing of the boundary between the self and the outside world. It is through the skin that we experience touch. Contact-comfort from our primary caregiver is a pivotal element of our survival as infants. If such touch was lacking, or conducted in an overly tentative, frightened, erratic, or unpredictable manner, we may have come to a level of suspicion of, and discomfort with, the boundary of our skin, the body's largest organ which is, in fact, an exposed part of the nervous system. How fitting, then, that we later turn to the cutting, burning, or picking of the skin to make sense of our pain.

Preoccupation with substances and/or behaviours is typically an intrinsic element of food and body image struggles. This preoccupation can come in many forms. Perhaps we are preoccupied with eating in general or with eating certain kinds of foods. Maybe we are preoccupied with starvation, or with other forms of body-related self-harm, like skin picking. Perhaps we are preoccupied with looking in the mirror, looking at celebrities' bodies in magazines, shopping for clothes that we believe will best flatter our bodies, or any manner of other possible manifestations.

Human beings come into this world already substance-dependent. The newborn is dependent on nourishment in the form of milk from either the breast or the bottle. Without this, the baby will die. Lack of milk is synonymous with death. Very early on, the teat or the nipple becomes linked in the infant's mind with satisfaction and safety, and its absence becomes linked with hunger, frustration, and fear, including the 'nameless dread' of death.

The mouth is the body part through which the desired satisfaction, in the form of milk, enters the human body. Psychoanalysts point to what they term the 'oral stage' of infant development, which typically takes place between the ages of birth and eighteen months. During the oral stage, the infant is focused on oral pleasures, such as sucking on the breast. Too much or too little gratification may result in an 'oral fixation', which tends to manifest as a preoccupation with oral activities like eating and drinking.

In the case of developmental trauma and attachment-based pain, preoccupations may arise later in life in an unconscious attempt to make sense of and 'undo' the psychological suffering experienced in infancy. Preoccupation is often likened to addiction, a term which has a plethora of different meanings for different people. It has also been suggested by some psychoanalysts, like Ernst Simmel, that addiction, as he terms it, serves to transform aggression towards the loved, yet hated object, which, in many cases, is a primary attachment figure—a notion linked to some of our explorations in earlier chapters. Related to this is the conceptualisation of preoccupations as an attempt to find soothing in a concrete form in the absence of good internalised objects, a concept we have also explored together.

In the post-World War period, psychoanalysts like Heinz Kohut began to look at addictive behaviours through the lens of a person's inability to self-soothe. Kohut believed that healthy development of the infant is dependent on having experienced consistent validation and affirmation of their identity. To describe this, Kohut used the term *mirroring*, denoting the recognition and response of a parent or caregiver to a child's needs, much like the *attunement* written about by John Bowlby, Mary Ainsworth and others. Without consistent validation of infantile needs, human beings can become highly vulnerable to the vicissitudes of their emotional states. Since harmony cannot be achieved in a state of high vulnerability within the self, *by* the self, the person seeks immediate relief in the form perhaps of food, substances, self-harm, and so on, resulting at some point in a cycle of preoccupation with the soothing object or behaviour.

Another layer to preoccupation is the issue of self-care. It has been suggested that people self-medicate with food, drugs, and other substances and practices because they lack the capacity for self-care. The capacity for self-care is a function of the ego, which develops during the infantile process of internalisation; the process of the infant internalising the comfort provided for by the caregiver within their own selves. It enables the infant to feel that they contain the immediacy and vitality of their primary caregiving relationship within themselves. Therefore, a person's preoccupation is adaptive. The compulsive behaviour or use of a substance (which could be food) is used to cope with seemingly intolerable emotions linked to seemingly intolerable experiences.

If we had the experience of our needs being met in infancy alongside consistent digestion of our emotional states by our primary caregiver, we would have been more likely to grow up with the tools to tolerate the fluctuations of our emotions. If we did not, we may go on to regularly have the experience of feeling overwhelmed by our emotions. Conversely, we might have the experience of feeling utterly numb, unable to sense our emotions at all. This can be equally as terrifying, if not more so. So, we reach for something outside of ourselves, either to terminate the seemingly unbearable feelings or to make us feel something. *Anything.* While we perhaps tend to more readily think of substances like drugs and alcohol when we think of addictive preoccupations, food or the denial of food are extremely common preoccupations, as are self-harm and body-focused, repetitive behaviours, like skin picking or pulling out one's hair (which are common correlates of BDD in particular).

Food is a desperate substance to be compulsively preoccupied with. This is because it is tangentially required for life. We cannot simply, therefore, empty our house and our lives of food and steer clear of it to be free of our compulsion. We must stare into the face of our preoccupation at every meal, grappling perhaps with how much food is too much and how little is too little. Perhaps we find ourselves hating and loving food simultaneously, splitting it both into the 'good object' and the 'bad object'. Perhaps we seem to spend almost as much time thinking about food as we do breathing. Perhaps we find images of food infiltrating even our dreams and nightmares. To add insult to already significant injury, the biology of the body can also be very strongly affected by food, particularly by certain foods and food groups.

You may recall from our discussion in Chapter Five how parallels can be drawn between our current eating habits and our early caregiving relationships. The types of food we choose can be intimately related to this. Breast milk is incredibly sweet, creamy, and high in fat. Some nutritionists say that the closest food to the nutritional composition of breast milk is ice cream, which seems highly plausible. Fat and sugar are two common food substances people can find themselves overeating. Sweet and crunchy foods can also be very compelling, as they additionally offer the visceral experience of chewing that we would have first experienced at the weaning stage of development.

Starvation itself can also be a compulsive behaviour. It can offer both emotional numbness (which can be experienced as soothing if we feel overwhelmed and/or confused by our emotions; if we feel hyper-aroused) and heightened physical sensations, such as pain, dizziness, and acute hunger (which can be experienced as soothing if we do not have a lived sense of our body; if we have poor interoceptive awareness and/or a tendency to dissociate from bodily sensations; if we feel hypo-aroused). Likewise, the act of self-induced vomiting can be both emotionally and physiologically compelling.

Let's take a closer look at a preoccupation with binge eating. This encompasses the sense of being compelled to eat, an experience of a loss of control over what is eaten and how much is eaten, and, commonly, feelings of guilt and shame during and/or after the consumption of food. It might also involve taking in more calories than the body needs. It may involve behaviours like thinking about food all the time (to the detriment of being able to concentrate on other things), eating rapidly, eating unpalatable foods (like under-ripe bananas or frozen bread), eating out of bins or other unusual places, eating until there is no food left in one's immediate vicinity, or eating in secret. Regardless, there will almost certainly be a loss of control. Some people describe losing a sense of the passage of time as they engage in a binge. Others describe the way the food seems to 'stuff down' their emotions. Others speak about how the food seems to engender a sense of aliveness in the body.

While compulsively eating to excess takes place in the present moment, as indeed everything does, the body-mind is rarely grounded in the present moment at these times. There may be partial or total dissociation, and/or a sense of being cut off from the body and its sensations. There may be a frenetic focus on the next moment, the next bite, the next swallow, or the next packet of food.

Compulsion cycles perpetuate when the body-mind is grounded outside of the present moment. This is usually because the present moment is felt to be too painful or too unbearable. Specifically, our thoughts suggest that the emotions rising in the present moment are too much to tolerate. So, we attempt to escape from the emotions, or to push them down, through the consumption or denial of food, self-induced vomiting, or whatever else it might be. These actions are, themselves, metaphors for our distress, as we explored together in the previous chapter.

Of course, we cannot escape our emotions. Life does not work that way. Our emotions are the energy set into motion because of various occurrences in our lives. They will not truly leave until they have completed their cycle—until they have been felt and until their story has been told.

Our emotions will keep knocking on our door, so to speak, until they have been experienced and listened to. We can only stuff them down with food for so long. As we munch our way through a box of breakfast cereal in one sitting, we may be temporarily numbed to our feeling of, say, loneliness or rejection. But these feelings will return after the binge-eating episode is over, typically in full-force, usually becoming even more virulently present than they were before. These feelings might lead us to the next box of cereal in a few hours' time, and so, the cycle becomes self-amplifying.

Biological aspects tend to contribute to these food-related, self-amplifying compulsion cycles. When we eat a large amount of food in a short period of time, our blood sugar levels are likely to spike considerably. This will then be followed by an inevitable blood sugar level 'crash', leading the body to seek more food to bring the blood sugar levels back up to a safe level. Similarly, eating too much of a singular food or food group can lead to vitamin and mineral deficiencies, prompting the body to seek the ingestion of more food to rebalance, say, potassium-sodium or zinc-copper levels. If we ingest a large amount of sodium in the form of salt, for example, the body will send signals that we need to drink or eat something water-dense and/or containing potassium to equilibrate. If we are not attuned to these nuances of our interoceptive signals, as many of us who engage in binge-eating, dieting, or starvation cycles are not, we may simply experience this as the drive to eat more. We may find ourselves eating compulsively, despite having eaten a large amount only an hour or two earlier.

The body will always strive to maintain homeostasis. In a healthy body, it will send out more insulin if the blood sugar levels are too high, release excessive sodium in the urine, get rid of excess copper through the faeces, bile, or skin, and so on. If you observe successfully individuated young children, you will notice that they intuitively know what to eat and in which amounts.

Some parents might postulate that their children would live on sweets, cakes, and ice cream alone if left to their own devices but this is simply not the case. If you provide a securely-attached young child with tables containing different categories of foods (e.g., fruits, vegetables, meats, grains, eggs, dairy, cakes, and sweets) they will indeed tend to go for the cakes and sweets first. This propensity is tied up with the biological drive to take in high-calorie food as insurance for future times of potential food scarcity. After some time, however, the child will begin to move over to the bread table, or the meat table. They may begin to actively choose the vegetables, despite the ongoing availability of chocolate and biscuits. You may remember a time when, as a child or an adult, you ate a lot of sweet stuff and later found yourself craving a plate of broccoli or a salad. The truth is, our body will communicate what it needs and strive towards homeostasis, overriding even the biological drive to take in high-calorie food.

We perhaps fear that if we allow ourselves to eat biscuits and cakes, for example, we will find ourselves eating almost nothing but biscuits and cakes. This fear is hugely unfounded. For a while, we might find ourselves eating biscuits to excess, just as most young children offered a range of food groups tend to overeat the sweet, high-calorie foods first. But in a perhaps surprisingly short space of time, we will naturally find ourselves moving away from the biscuits and towards the nutrients in other foods which our bodies are now lacking.

We often link the ingestion of certain foods not only with feelings of temporary satisfaction and emotional numbing but also, on the other side of the coin, shame and guilt. This is a painful combination. You eat the biscuit and the seeking energy is momentarily gratified. Compulsion leads you to eat the next biscuit, then the next, then the next. Your heart races. Your shaking hands can hardly get the biscuits into your mouth rapidly enough. Soon enough, the whole packet is gone. Guilt and shame wash over you. Still, your body is not satisfied. And, still, the difficult emotions continue to press upon your heart.

If we were deeply tuned into our interoceptive signals, as typically-developing and securely-attached young children are, and had no need to stuff down our emotions, we would later find ourselves digging into a protein-rich meal or a plate piled high with vegetables. Instead, perhaps, we forbid ourselves from eating anything else that day, having ingested the whole packet of biscuits. An hour or two later, the blood sugar level in the body plummets. Perhaps we find ourselves bingeing again or perhaps we push through this, feeling terrible physically, only to repeat the cycle at some point later that day or week. Likely, our thoughts then suggest this is completely our fault. Thoughts like: *I should have more self-control, I am greedy, I should have been able to stop myself* may subsequently arise, leading to further guilt and shame.

We find ourselves, again, at the notion of free will and choice, and at the concept of identity. We feel shame and guilt because we believe the 'I' we take ourselves to be is responsible for overeating. We have usually divorced this sense of 'I' from the myriad of literally millions of other factors that 'caused' the overeating to take place: Elements of our caregiver's history, our own life history, our attachment patterns, our emotions and the root of these emotions, the availability of the food, our biology, and so on, ad infinitum. Each of these elements, and many more besides, played an irrevocable part in the act of overeating the food. Given these myriad of factors, which would be too numerous to name, we cannot lay the blame for any episode of overeating on any one thing. We cannot, indeed, lay the blame for anything at the feet of any one thing or phenomena. As Yogi Bhajan said, *'Every sequence has a consequence.'* When a sequence is set into motion, a consequence organically plays itself out. This sequence is likely to have started even before our lifetime. Taking some responsibility for our actions is very useful but ascribing guilt and shame to them is not.

This may sound nihilistic. It may even sound terrifying, since it seems to suggest the body-mind has no control and no 'say' in anything it does or anything that unravels in its life. At the level of the body-mind, this would appear to be true. Thankfully, the body-mind is not who we are. We are Freedom itself. Freedom is, by its very nature, free. So, we *do* have the freedom to 'choose', just not perhaps in the way we think.

Let us return to our example of eating a whole packet of biscuits. In part, your biology 'made you do it'. In part, your emotional experience 'made you do it'. In part, the availability of food in modern society 'made you do it', and so on. All of these are true, perhaps, at the level of the body-mind and, tangentially, none of these are true at the level of the true Self—of unadulterated Freedom—which is who you intrinsically are. When we identify ourselves as the body-mind, life plays itself out accordingly. When we identify ourselves as the *awareness* of the body-mind, phenomena such as eating a whole packet of biscuits do not seem to happen. Freedom does not need to eat a whole packet of biscuits in order to escape difficult sensations and emotions. Freedom is not afraid of difficult sensations and emotions. Freedom permits all experiences, welcoming difficult sensations and emotions as opportunities for the body-mind to remember its wholeness. Freedom invites the cycle of feeling an emotion, expressing an emotion, receiving soothing for an emotion and the emotion leaving or assimilating.

Where does this leave us then, practically, in terms of moving beyond compulsions like overeating? What can we do about it?

At the level of the body-mind, we might be able to train our minds and our bodies not to eat the whole packet of biscuits. We might 'update' the environment by keeping biscuits out of the house. We might 'update' the behaviour by doing some yoga when we feel the urge to binge, immersing ourselves in a creative pursuit like drawing or sculpting, calling up a friend, or crunching on carrot sticks instead. All of these can be extremely useful strategies and, as someone who has used all of them and many others besides, I am certainly not being disparaging about them in any way. They can go a long way to reduce the suffering of the body-mind. Here are some other very practical examples that were particularly supportive for me:

- Taking a few long, deep breaths when the urge to binge emerges. Connect with the heart centre and ask the soul what it is aching for. Listen to the soul and respond to its yearnings.
- Spending some time engaged in long, deep breathing while feeling into the emotions before eating/not eating.
- Resisting 'making up rules' about eating in terms of food types and times for eating, and instead attempting to tune into the body (see next point).
- Trying to 'listen' to the body and discern what it is craving physiologically. For example, asking yourself: *Do my blood sugar levels need raising? My blood pressure? Is my body looking for a specific nutrient?* For example, I found that my craving for chocolate was often a need for magnesium and/or dampening down feelings of sadness.
- Including a source of protein with every meal to keep the blood sugar levels stable.
- Eating a variety of vegetation sources to ensure that the body receives the macro and micro nutrients it needs.
- Including a bit of unrefined sea salt in meals to keep your blood pressure stable (if it tends to be low).
- Avoiding caffeine, which tends to kick-off a blood-sugar

rollercoaster.

- Keeping the body adequately hydrated.
- Refraining from going down the shop aisles known to contain the foods you tend to binge on when you are feeling emotionally 'rocky'.
- Eating at regular intervals during the day (meals and snacks) to negate becoming overwhelmed by hunger.
- Munching on crunchy foods like raw carrots when the urge to binge (and possibly purge) feels almost overwhelming (only after eating an adequate amount of a meal or snack beforehand, of course).
- Practicing yoga, engaging in creative pursuits, going for a walk etc. when feelings of anxiety about a meal or the urge to binge emerge.
- Imagining your body as the body of someone you love when you feel like skipping a meal or you begin to agonise over what you should eat. Try asking yourself what you would feed the person you love, and feed yourself accordingly.
- When deciding what to eat, asking yourself: *What would love choose?*
- Wearing clothes that are not tight around the stomach and thighs, so there is less discomfort and related fear if they feel tighter after eating. Throwing clothes away if they no longer fit or do not feel comfortable in any way.
- Throwing away your bathroom scales.
- Accepting that it can sometimes take the body a while to feel full and to assimilate the food. Many people who binge and/or diet to excess come to struggle with degrees of reactive hypoglycaemia. This can mean that eating makes you feel tired and shaky. This can be improved by including a source of protein in each meal and snack. It can also really help to sit at the table for up to half an hour after eating while breathing slowly and deeply, thereby

giving time and space for any uncomfortable physical sensations to pass.

It is quite possible that the body needs very specific things if we have spent any time restricting our nutritional intake or engaging in binge-eating episodes. There is not a 'one-size-fits-all' diet, as far as I can tell. There has been a recent explosion, hugely through the Internet and social media, of innumerable possible diets which claim to be the perfect recipe for human health and ideal weight. No diet could ever uphold such a promise, since every human body has a unique nutritional history, metabolism, balance of blood sugar and nutrients, and so on. It amazes me just how many diets are out there, each making totally oppositional claims. One expounds a view that high-fat, low-carbohydrate foods are the Holy Grail, while another berates the presence of any fat in the diet, while another implores the need for a high proportion of the diet to be carbohydrate-based. Whichever possibility, there is a diet with a name for it, and certainly a high-profit business behind it. Clean eating has become a concerning and prevalent one, with rules that sound uncomfortably similar (read 'the same') as the diagnosis of orthorexia.

It is possible to become compulsively preoccupied with dieting (as a wise person once said, 'Do not trust a word with the letters D-I-E in it!') or with a specific way of eating. It is common to hear that people end up replacing one preoccupation for another. This can also happen when we try, through the sheer force of will, to change our compulsive behaviours. This seems to happen because the underlying emotional pain, which harbours a story that is begging to be understood and told, is still present. It happens because a trauma-cycle, somewhere along the line, has not completed itself and, thus, the related emotions have become lodged in the body somehow. Perhaps it feels safer to exercise to excess than to eat to excess, but the former is no less of a compulsion. And still, the emotional turmoil continues to stagnate.

This is by no means suggesting that we are powerless against our preoccupations and compulsions. Quite the opposite. In fact, we are the power itself.

When we rediscover who we truly are and hold this discovery within our awareness, every action will be experienced as an expression of love. From this place, bingeing is very unlikely to happen, as there is no identification or resistance to the perceived difficult emotions that the bingeing had been attempting to stuff down. The invitation is to take our stand as Love, witness the emotions as they arise, and fully allow them to be there, welcoming them as golden shadows and necessary expressions of the Love we are. Emotions in the form of sensations arise and we permit them and feel into them fully. The emotions take their opportunity to tell their story and then depart. We have no need to stuff the emotions down with food or starvation because we have no fear of them. We recognise our emotions as holders of our story and invitations to our wholeness.

We are the open, aware space within which all emotions arise and dissolve. We turn to compulsions like overeating or starving ourselves in order to push our emotions away, believing that we cannot bear them. Who is this 'I' who cannot bear these emotions? Can you find that 'I'? Look and you will discover that you are already free.

Our experience might have been that of living as a prisoner of food, or whatever else we are preoccupied with. The truth is there is no prison, nor are there any jail keepers. The truth is that we are liberated, and always have been.

It is possible to come to a place where food is experienced as just food. Hunger is felt, food is sought and taken in, physical satisfaction is interocepted, and the body-mind goes about its day. No agonising, no guilt, no shame. No feeling of I shouldn't have eaten that or spending interminable minutes or hours thinking about what will be eaten for the next meal. Eating can become as natural and as painless as regular breathing. Imagine that.

These days, when I notice my thoughts turning towards over- or under-eating, I sit quietly, sink down into my heart centre and openly welcome any sensations and emotions that are present. When I embrace and fully feel into these emotions and allow myself to express them in whichever way feels natural, the drive to overeat or under-eat melts away. This is the freedom to choose at the level of the true Self. The true Self has already made its choice and this choice is always based in freedom and love. When our resistance falls away, the choice of the true Self can be felt and is taken. This is an organic process. A process of ease. A natural unfolding.

The invitation is to actively take our stand as Awareness/ Freedom/Love, moment-by-moment, when thoughts or feelings related to the compulsion cycle begin to arise. There is a noticing of the emotion, an active welcoming of the emotion, a diving into the body-based sensations of the emotion, an expression of the emotion, and then, time for the body to respond naturally with tears, sleep, laughter, stillness, or whatever it might be. In the early days of beginning this practice, it might be that this cycle is repeated many times each day as the emotions work their way to the surface.

As we assume the position of the witnessing presence and this position becomes embedded in the experience of the body-mind, it might be that we notice our emotions more quickly and that the cycle begins to flow more effortlessly, rapidly, and seamlessly. Eventually, it might be that our emotions flow through us so freely that the cycle of noticing, embracing, expressing and assimilating becomes instinctive and there is no longer any conscious intention or action attached to it. When this happens, not only do the shame and guilt attached to eating fall away; so, too, does the need to overeat, under-eat, weigh the body, use clothes to hide the body, over-exercise, and so on.

Freedom has no interest in any of these things. Who you truly are has no interest in any of these things.

Food Meditation

Place an item of food in front of you that you tend to not allow yourself to eat and/or typically feel guilty about eating. Close your eyes and take a few long, deep breaths. Fill your lungs from the bottom-up with each inhalation and draw your abdomen back towards your spine at the end of each exhalation, emptying your lungs completely. Take a few moments to relax each part of your body in turn, starting with your toes and finishing at the crown of your head.

When you sense a feeling of relaxation in your body, slowly open your eyes and witness the food item in front of you. Notice any reactions or sensations that show up in your body as you place your attention on the food. Feel into these sensations without judgement, allowing them to be there just as they are.

Sink back into the very deepest part of yourself, turning your awareness around to focus on itself. Place your awareness on Awareness. Spend a few seconds like this and then return your awareness and your attention to the food. Continue like this, shifting your focus from the food to Awareness, to the sense of 'I' within you, and then back to the food again.

Merge these two experiences and witness the food from your 'I-ness'. Witness the food in the space of love and freedom that you intrinsically are.

Pick up the food and hold it in your hands. Notice that the sense of touching the food arises in your awareness: In who you are. Bring the food slowly to your nose. Smell the food from this place of 'I-ness'. Notice that the smell of the food arises in the same place as the sensation of touching the food. Both arise in a witnessing presence, which is closer than close. Allow your tongue to emerge. Taste the food. Notice that the sensation of tasting arises in the same place as the smell and feel of the food. They all take place within you, within Awareness.

Go ahead and take a bite of the food. Fully enter the sensations of taste, smell, texture, and swallowing. Welcome any reactions that show up in the body, noticing that these emerge in the same place as the tasting and smelling. It is all the same experience. It is all Awareness being aware of itself.

Eat your food, welcoming fully any reactions that show up, including fear and resistance. These, too, are modulations of Awareness, of Love. How could Love be threatened by anything, least of all itself?

Finish by sending love to the food, the hands that harvested or created it, and your body for taking it in and turning it into energy to keep the body-mind alive and able to feel, think, move, and connect. Bless yourself. Give yourself a hug. Allow any emotions to surface and play themselves out. Be kind and compassionate to yourself.

To finish this chapter, I would like to offer you a list of possible questions you could ask yourself when deciding which food and drinks to nourish yourself with at any given time. It could be useful to take five minutes when you notice you are feeling hungry to ask yourself some or all of these questions. Or, if you are not yet in touch with your hunger and fullness signals (don't worry, this usually takes time!) you can do this before a designated mealtime or at a time when you feel you may be hungry. Take a few deep, mindful breaths and feel into each question with your body sensations. Notice your gut reaction to each question. Your body will let you know the answer if you listen, perhaps in the form of a physical sensation, such as a lurch in the stomach, an ache in the throat, tingling, a 'whoosh' of desire, a contraction of the muscles, or a 'premonition' of how the food may make you feel.

If possible, avoid engaging too much with your thoughts as you do this, focusing instead on the sensations of the body. Your thoughts are likely to offer all sorts of excuses which, in my experience, are rarely in line with the truth. For example, you might hear your body asking for fish, but your thoughts might jump in with all sorts of excuses, like, *you don't have any fish at home, you don't eat fish because you are a vegan!* and many other possibilities besides. Your thoughts favour familiarity alongside their propensity to polarise everything. The invitation is to allow your thoughts to wash over you as you tune deeply into what your body wants and needs.

I hope you will find this list of questions helpful.

- What sensations can I detect in my body right now? *(E.g., shakiness, pain, movement, fullness, emptiness, a fast heartbeat, an elevated breathing rate, or relaxed/contracted muscles.)*
- What needs might each of these sensations be pointing to? *(E.g., are my blood sugar levels low? Does my body require physical nourishment? Are there emotional needs present, such as the need for connection, closeness, and soothing?)*
- Where in my body do I feel my hunger? Is it in my stomach? *(This may be more likely to be physical hunger.)* Or is it in my chest, throat, or mouth? *(This may be more likely to be emotional hunger.)*
- Which foods are coming to mind? *(Take each food one-by-one and give it your full attention.)* As I place this food in my awareness, what bodily sensations are coming up? Are these attached to any memories or emotions? How do I imagine I will feel after eating this food, physically and emotionally? *(Repeat these questions as you place each food that comes to mind in your awareness. Refrain from buying into anything your thoughts might suggest.)*
- *(Imagine each of the foods that come to mind spread out on a table in front of you.)* Which food seems to draw my interest most strongly? Why do I think this might be? *(Tune into your connection with your stomach.)* What would my stomach choose? *(Tune into your whole body.)* Which of these foods does my body yearn for in this present moment?
- *(Imagine yourself twenty minutes after eating the food you felt drawn to.)* How does my body feel? What is my

predominant emotional state? Considering my answers to these questions, would this be the optimal food to choose in this moment? *(If the answer is 'no', keep moving through the foods on your virtual table until you find one that best supports your future self, both emotionally and physically.)*

After you have finished asking yourself these questions, imagine your future self, one hour from now. Sit beside your future self in your mind's eye. Which food does it seem to suggest? Listen to the reasons why. Thank your future self.

You can also consult trusted others in your mind's eye if you find this helpful. I often consult my granddad, who died many years ago. It was his 'advice' that led me to begin eating nuts after avoiding fats for many years.

A Note on *Ahimsa*

A core yogic principle is *Ahimsa*, meaning 'non-violence'. *Ahimsa* begins at home. We can practise *Ahimsa* in whatever food choices we make. This means listening to our bodies and lovingly providing them with whatever they biologically yearn for. I find it impossible to believe that human beings were designed to feel hungry all the time, which is how we might feel if we restrict our diets and deny ourselves of the sensation of satiation. We can demonstrate non-violence to ourselves by filling our stomachs with nourishing, sustaining foods, thereby stimulating the stretch receptors and feelings of satiation and energy. This will look differently for each of us, depending on our constitution, dieting history, and so on. We have more important things to do during our time on this Earth than to be perpetually consumed by feelings of hunger. Fuelling our bodies lovingly is true *Ahimsa*, whatever those food requirements are for each of our bodies. Eating to our satisfaction provides us with the energy and headspace to shine the light we were born to shine in this world.

Chapter Twelve

Listen to the Body 'Speak'

Western philosophy and science most typically position the body as both separate and inferior to the mind. The mind/body split, as epitomised by Rene Descartes' exaltation, *'I think; therefore, I am,'* would appear to be rooted in the Enlightenment quest for rational knowledge and absolute truth, for realism, over relativist ontological conceptualisations of the world. Other Western philosophers, such as Maurice Merleau-Ponty, theorised that the ability to perceive (sentience) can only be experienced in and through the body; thus, challenging the mind/body split. Others have gone further, placing the body hierarchically above the mind, as captured in philosopher Baruch Spinoza's statement, *'I feel; therefore, I am.'*

Spinoza understood the body as being inextricable from perception. Essentially, when we try to extrapolate our sensory experience of the world from the body, we come away empty-handed. The world is brought to us through our senses, which are brought to us through our bodies.

If all goes well, the newborn infant is laid skin-to-skin, heart-to-heart with their mother/father/primary caregiver. This, and other early attachment experiences, are body-to-body experiences. These experiences take place pre-verbally and, thus, are stored implicitly, within our procedural memory. Procedural memory is a type of implicit, unconscious memory concerned with the process of retrieving the information necessary to perform learned tasks. It encompasses all automatic performances, unconscious dispositions, and nonverbal habits of behaviour. Declarative (explicit) memory, on the other hand, records single experiences for later recall.

Psychiatrist Bessel van der Kolk and others have suggested

that our procedural memory is likely to be dominated by emotional and impressionistic information, and is accessible only by performance (i.e., by being 'lived out' through the body). Thus, we may not have a verbal memory of the awkwardness of our caregiver's embrace in infancy, but our procedural memory will 'keep the score', perhaps manifesting in a stiffness in our limbs, spontaneous withdrawal at the touch of another, arms that stay primarily by our sides, as opposed to reaching out as an initial response to an embrace, and so on.

Our implicit memory system contains stored patterns of body-based, emotional interactions which are unconsciously activated by subtle situational cues, such as facial expressions, prosody of voice, gestures, and so on. Trying to understand, move through, and assimilate our experiences using thought and reason alone, therefore, is unlikely to reach our preverbal experiences since they are stored in the sensations, reactions, and movements of the body.

It is interesting that clinical guidelines, such as the NICE Guidelines in the UK, tend to emphasise 'talking cures' and medication for appearance-focused identity struggles like eating disorders and BDD. These struggles play themselves out in the body, are based in the body, and relate to implicit memories stored within the body. I would assert, therefore, that the 'cure' is more likely to exist and take place in and through the body at a level deeper than verbalisation alone.

The body is a source of information about the experiences we 'cannot remember' in the form of explicit memory. The body will 'speak' of our early pain whether we listen or not. If we actively listen, however, our story has a chance to be told. We have a chance to assimilate this story. We have a chance to move on.

The language of the body emerges through the breath, contraction and relaxation of the muscles, digestion, blood flow, temperature, movement, and much more. We will now take some time to go through some of the ways in which our body tells our story, looking also at ways in which we can use this body-narrative to hear and assimilate our story and, thus, our emotional pain.

Breath

The breath is the signature of all our emotional states. We tend to breathe in cycles, breathing for two hours predominantly through the left nostril, followed by two hours breathing predominantly through the right nostril. Breathing through the left nostril is calming to the nervous system, while breathing through the right nostril is stimulating and invigorating. We can alter our nostril predominance by taking long, deep breaths through the alternative nostril for twenty-six breath cycles. If we wish to enjoy relaxed sleep, we might like to try sleeping on our right side; thus, allowing us to predominantly breathe out of the left nostril while tangentially inviting fluid to drain from the heart.

It is estimated that eighty per cent of the Western world are predominantly chest-breathers (thoracic breathers). They breathe primarily into their upper chest, failing to use the full capacity of their lungs to take in and expel air. You can check to see if you are a chest-breather by placing one hand on your abdomen and the other on your chest. Spread your fingers so that the upper hand covers the full expanse of your chest, up to your clavicle. Breathe normally and notice which parts of the body move as you breathe, and in which order they move. Predominantly chest-breathers will find that their chest expands as they inhale and deflates as they exhale (or deflates as they inhale and expands as they exhale, if they are breathing paradoxically), with little movement in their abdominal area. They are breathing with the top section of their lungs. To ascertain that this is indeed your natural breath pattern, ask a trusted other to observe your breath at rest and/or during sleep, when you are not aware, therefore, negating the possible impact of your awareness on the alteration of your breath.

The upper ten per cent of our lungs transports less than six millilitres of oxygen per minute, in comparison to the lower ten per cent of our lungs, which transports more than forty millilitres of oxygen per minute. Therefore, the lower part of the lungs is about six to seven times more effective in oxygen transportation than the top part of the lungs, due to a richer blood supply. If we breathe primarily from our upper chest, the lower layers of the lungs (which are more valuable in oxygen transportation) get less, if any, fresh air (which means less oxygen supply). This results in reduced oxygenation of blood in the lungs.

In addition, when we breathe primarily from our upper chest, we fail to stimulate the cleansing work of the lymph system, which increases the rate of the elimination of toxins from visceral organs by about fifteen times. This is significant, as the lymph system has no pump of its own. The lymph nodes connected to the stomach, kidney, liver, pancreas, spleen, large and small colons, and other vital organs are located just under the diaphragm, comprising over sixty per cent of all lymph nodes in total. Breathing, therefore, is the main way in which we remove waste products from our vital organs. Chest-breathing, therefore, can result in stagnation in the lymph system, causing the accumulation of waste products in vital organs.

Chest-breathing typically has an emotional base and emotional consequences, in addition to these physiological ramifications. Early life experiences can lead to a chest-breathing predominance. When our caregivers are attuned to us, we are provided with a sense of safety that manifests in long, relaxed breathing, utilising the full capacity of our lungs. Conversely, if our early attachment relationships are unpredictable, disregarding, and/or frightening in any way, our bodies can guard themselves in the form of contracted muscles and sympathetic or dorsal vagal activation. The movement of the diaphragm, which is itself a muscle, becomes constricted and the breath remains in the top part of the chest. In a sorry case of circularity, this shallow chest-breathing further stimulates the sympathetic nervous system, resulting in a perpetuating lived experience of danger.

Another typical breathing pattern that emerges from early experiences of attachment-based, developmental trauma is paradoxical or reverse-belly breathing. In paradoxical breathing, the abdomen is drawn in on the inhalation and expands outwards on the exhalation. Again, this breathing pattern is often both a reflection of sympathetic arousal and a stimulator of it. We can discern this pattern by placing a hand, with fingers spread, on the abdomen and noticing when and how the navel moves inwards and outwards as we breathe normally. Again, it can be helpful to enlist the support of a trusted other to confirm this, as the very act of drawing our attention to our breathing can unconsciously alter it.

A sense of safety within the body is typically displayed through breath that utilises the full capacity of the lungs, with the abdomen moving outwards on the inhalation and dropping back towards the spine on the exhalation.

Two exercises are offered below for noticing and gently altering the breath and the sense of safety in the body; thus, bringing the physiological and emotional states within the window of tolerance.

Exercise One: The Breath as Information

Place one hand on your abdomen and the other on your chest, with the fingers of your upper hand spreading to reach your clavicle. Close your eyes or cast your gaze downwards if this helps you focus. Breathe normally and notice the movement of your hands as you do so. Notice whether your abdomen or chest moves first when you inhale and in which direction it moves (such as outwards, inwards, upwards, or downwards). Now, notice whether your abdomen or chest moves first when you exhale and in which direction it moves. Apply no judgement. Simply notice.

Continue to place your awareness on your breath and ask yourself what its pattern might be communicating. Consider that shallow breath that takes place mostly in the upper chest may be communicating a level of stress, anxiety, or tension. It could be communicating that there was a time in your life when you didn't feel safe and secure. Notice that it is not necessary to find an explicit memory of this time, but rather, to feel into the sensation of your breath and the message it is delivering. Take as much time as you need to stay with your breath, diving into its sensations and impressions without attempting to distract yourself from them. Stay with any emotions that emerge with or following these sensations. Laugh if you feel moved to laugh. Cry if you feel moved to cry.

Exercise Two: Full Breathing

Having spent some time feeling into the sensations and emotions linked to your usual breathing pattern, feel free to begin to deepen your breathing. As you breathe in, expand your abdomen outwards, filling your lungs from the bottom up, expanding your abdomen, then your chest area, then your clavicle. When you feel you have reached your full lung capacity, take another small sip of air. Notice the pause at the top of the inhalation. Slowly begin to exhale, emptying first the top part of your lungs (your clavicle area drops back), then the middle part of your lungs (your chest area drops back), then the lower part of your lungs (your abdomen drops back). Allow your abdomen to consciously drop back towards your spine. At the end of the exhalation, lightly pull up on your navel to completely empty your lungs of air. Notice the pause at the end of the exhalation before the next inhalation begins.

As before, stay with the sensations in your body as you practise this breathing pattern. Notice any resistance and breathe into this also. Feel into the resistance, allowing any sensations to surface. Welcome any sensations with a full embrace and permit any emotions to emerge in whichever way they spontaneously arise.

Slowing down our breath can have an immense impact on our brains, nervous system, and our emotional, psychological, and spiritual state. If we reduce our breath to eight breath cycles (one full inhalation and exhalation) per minute, we enter the relaxation state. If we reduce this further, to four breath cycles per minute, we come into the meditation state. At one breath cycle per minute, we are in the yogic state (union of the finite with the infinite). We do this by inhaling for twenty seconds, lightly suspending our breath for twenty seconds and exhaling for twenty seconds. We can build up to this gradually, perhaps starting with eight-second cycles and increasing each cycle over time with patience and self-compassion.

Posture

Our posture, in many ways, could be said to gradually become the epitomised 'statue' of our cumulative experiences. The way we hold ourselves can harbour a plethora of information—not only about our experiences but also how we have made sense of them. Merleau-Ponty described how the body-memory plays a special part in changing a person's corporeal and intercorporeal experiences into implicitly effective predispositions, including how we stand, walk, sit, lay down, speak, use gestures, and so on.

In a sense, the situations and actions we have experienced in our histories become 'fused together', as Thomas Fuchs puts it, thereby generating a habit structure. This includes well-practised motion sequences, repeated perceived body schemas, and forms of actions and interactions which comprise implicit bodily knowledge and skill. Prior to being able to reflect on what we are communicating through our speech and gestures, our body expresses itself, while, at the same time, reacting to the impressions of others. This can be very subtle and highly nuanced. This intercorporeality forms a system through which, from childhood onwards, forms of bodily interaction are established and continually updated. Thus, with every interaction, our intercorporeality may shift and amend slightly or, at times, even dramatically. This may take place at the conscious level but may also take place—whether primarily or completely—at the unconscious level.

Freud famously stated that symptoms have both a meaning and a function. We could conceive of the lived expressions of our body-memory as 'symptoms' of our early life experiences. We might then find ourselves becoming curious about the meanings and functions they are serving to communicate and emit. Let us take the example of hurting our leg. We instinctively curl the body over and reach out the arms to hold, soothe, and protect the leg. Here, instinctual patterns of survival come into play in addition to body-memory based on previous experiences of pain. The posture we adopt is referred to by Fuchs as a 'relieving posture'. Avoidance behaviour is implicit within this relieving posture. We are avoiding not only the pain but also, potentially, the memory of that which *caused* the pain—the injuring event. It could be argued that avoidance is implicit in each of our spontaneous postural behaviours in some way or another. Over time, these behaviours can become 'frozen postures'. For example, walking with perpetually-stooped shoulders might be indicative of repeated experiences of shame. It could be that what is potentially threatening in the environment—such as the shaming caregiver—is no longer consciously experienced. Rather, it is solely experienced unconsciously through the avoidance reactions and postures of the body.

Merleau-Ponty described how the unconscious has a life of its own, selecting what will be admitted to official existence and creating detours around the thoughts and feelings we resist. Therefore, rather than a 'not-knowing', he suggests that the unconscious is perhaps better understood as unacknowledged, unformulated knowledge that we are defended against and that we believe we cannot tolerate. He goes on to describe how what is repressed becomes like a phantom limb for an amputee; a bodily capacity continues in the amputee through the sense of a phantom limb, which is no longer congruent with the present reality of their body; in the same way in which a lived impression continues in the body of the emotion or experience we have cut ourselves off from.

In this way, the current body and the habitual body come into conflict with one another. Similarly, a repressed experience (and its associated thoughts and feelings) which has been avoided— and, therefore, not dealt with—overlays and conflicts with the current experience; thus, imprisoning the person in *'a past which is still present,'* to use Fuchs' words. What is repressed is hidden from sight and held within the body. It lives not as an explicit memory but as an implicit 'phantom'. Bodily patterns of behaviour can also represent a past which is still present. These implicit body-memories may also underlie the repetition compulsion, wherein we tend to repeat and become drawn back into similar patterns of painful situations, experiences, and relationships in an unconscious bid to resolve them. Appearance-focused identity struggles seem to operate within this pattern. We repeatedly gaze in the mirror, binge and purge, starve ourselves, spend innumerable hours at the gym, and so on—despite knowing, somehow, that these behaviours never ultimately result in the peace and happiness we crave. Perhaps the attraction is largely at the unconscious, implicit, body-memory level, as the body leans towards what it is embroiled in, recognises, resonates with, and 'knows' all too well.

Exercise Three: Listening to Your Posture

Imagine pressing a 'pause' button as you sit here. Become still, without changing anything about your posture and without adding any additional tension to your muscles or joints. Start at your feet, noticing how they are positioned. Be sure to notice without judgement. Next, notice the positioning of your legs, paying attention to your ankle and knee joints. Move up to your hips, offering your full attention to any looseness or tightness. Notice whether your hips sit parallel to each other or whether one is higher and/or more open than the other. Move up through your abdomen and chest area, noticing any openness or collapse. Next, notice how your spine is positioned. Pay attention to your spine as if were the most fascinating thing in the world. Take your time with this. Next, move to your shoulders, before turning your attention to the positioning of your hands, delving into the position of each finger in turn. How are your wrists positioned? Your elbows? Finally, notice how you are holding first your neck and then your head. Is your chin tucked in or does it reach forwards over your chest? Is your head tilted to one side? What about the elements of your face? Is your tongue 'stuck' to the roof of your mouth or is it loose in your lower palate? Are your eyes cast downwards, upwards, or straight ahead?

After scanning through the position of each body part, sit for a while in the awareness of what you have uncovered. Which elements of your posture particularly captivated your attention? Stay with these, delving into any physical sensations that accompany them. Allow any related memories or emotions to emerge without censorship. Allow that part of your body to 'speak'.

Practise this exercise in the same way in other positions, such as lying down or walking if you are able. In the case of walking, the 'pause' button does not terminate the act of walking but, rather, stops any alteration of the walking pattern. Simply continue to walk as you were before, bringing your attention to each element of your posture in turn, with each step.

Exercise Four: Postural Healing

Stay with the element of your posture that has particularly captivated your attention. Immerse your awareness in the physical sensations and any memories and feelings that emerge from this. Refrain from trying to make sense of them cognitively. Simply stay with their lived, sensation-based experience. If the sensations or the accompanying emotions or memories begin to feel frightening or overwhelming, breathe into them. As Winston Churchill so wisely said, 'If you are going through hell, keep going.' The light is within the darkness, not outside it. If you feel yourself beginning to dissociate, ground yourself in the physical environment by opening your eyes. Notice the visual phenomena in your present environment. Also notice sounds and smells. Perhaps take a few moments to recall times in your life when you have felt supported and safe. Who was there with you when you experienced this? Invite a sense of support and safety into your current experience. Immerse yourself in this feeling. When you feel ready, you can return to your practice. Return your attention to the sensations related to an element of your posture, bringing the sense of support and safety with you.

Allow any expressive behaviours to spontaneously emerge.

Take time after your practice to be kind to yourself. You might feel the need to rest, take a nap, go for a walk in nature, take some time to journal, or any manner of other things. Your body will let you know what it needs.

The Spontaneous 'Talk' of the Body

We have described how we can provide space and invite the body to speak to us. Often, however, the body will speak to us spontaneously as we go about our everyday lives. This can feel very confusing at times and can take us by surprise. It can also be very much unconscious. We do not necessarily consciously notice that our body is speaking to us but, rather, find ourselves engaging in behaviours to avoid the unconscious sensation-based messages. Food-related behaviours are one example of this in the context of appearance-focused identity struggles. For example, we might find ourselves reaching into the cupboard to devour a whole loaf of bread without any conscious notion of what triggered us to do so. Yet, an event or sequence of events will have triggered implicit memories stored within the body, leading up to this moment. Such events can be as subtle as a dream we had the night prior but do not remember, the scent of a passing stranger that smells a bit like the perfume our primary caregiver used to wear, or a piece of music whose sequence of notes is similar to a song we heard during a difficult period of our early history and so on.

Therefore, it is often very challenging to pinpoint the triggers for our sense of discomfort and resultant expressive behaviour. This is especially difficult because we are unlikely to have explicit memories to map on to them. Instead, the invitation is most typically one of trusting our body-based sensations and expressive behaviours as messengers to a past our bodies remember but our cognition does not.

When we have uncomfortable body-sensations or find ourselves engaging in soothing behaviours we cannot find a conscious trigger for, it can be helpful to pause for a moment and return to the exercises in this chapter. Pause and pay attention to your breath. Pause and pay attention to your posture. Dive into the sensations. Allow the associated feelings and emotions to emerge. Allow their release, however the body spontaneously moves towards releasing them. If you are in a very public place or in the middle of something that would make an extended pause difficult, perhaps take a few mindful breaths and commit to taking some time later in the day to return to this sensation or behaviour. For example, before returning home to binge-eat in order to shove the emotion down, take some time to complete the exercises laid out in this chapter. Seeking out and practising a Kundalini kriya or meditation before engaging in the act of bingeing/purging etc. can also be incredibly transformative. You can find hundreds of kriyas and meditations in the Library of Teachings located at www.libraryofteachings.com. Go to the search bar, select 'kriyas' from the drop-down menu and type in a key word (i.e., *fear, hunger, loneliness*) to find a kriya and/ or meditation to support you. You are also welcome to access the Kundalini Celestial Communications I have recorded for my YouTube Channel, which you can access at www.youtube.com/c/PointofLight.

Scheduling time each day for practices like these is a tremendous act of self-care. Telling yourself that you are 'too busy' and 'cannot fit it in' is, of course, avoidance. We can all find twenty minutes in our day and will typically find that taking such time out of our day will mean:

- The rest of our day unfolds more smoothly.
- We are less distracted during the rest of our day, therefore becoming more productive (and thereby actually saving time).
- We are less likely to engage in self-defeating expressive behaviours, which take time out of our day and typically ignite distress and shame.

Sometimes, listening to our body in these ways will provide us with messages we (think we) do not want to hear. It is more accurate to say they may provide us with messages *our false selves* do not want to hear. Our true Selves are always open to the truth, however painful this might be. We may have been running from these messages for many years, or perhaps even our whole lives. Therefore, it is not uncommon to find ourselves engaging in repeated distraction-based behaviours, particularly when we are coming 'close' to feeling and hearing the hidden experiences stored within our body. The closer we come, the further we might subsequently retract. This, in and of itself, can become a pattern.

At these times of retraction, there is an invitation to embed our lived-sense in our true Selves, which are open to the truth in every moment, even if, on a surface level, this might completely shatter our current reality or seemingly tear our lives apart. Our true Selves understand that our identity is not the body-mind and has everything to do with our transpersonal, love-imbued nature. It is of no worry to the true Self that the assimilation of a painful experience may change the personal body-mind self in some way. On the contrary, the true Self leans towards this freedom in every moment of our lives.

One way to embed ourselves in the true Self is to practise self-enquiry. This practice shall be the focus of our next and final chapter.

Chapter Thirteen

Practise Self-Enquiry and Remember Who You Truly Are

We have explored aspects of the practice of self-enquiry as we have moved through these pages together. It describes, at its root, a manner of exploration within which we delve into the truth of who we are.

Let us begin our deeper exploration by writing down a list of sentences beginning with the words 'I am'. Allow yourself to free-associate, without hesitation or overthinking. Write down at least three sentences beyond the point when your thoughts suggest that you can think of no more. For example:

I am Nicole.
I am thirty-five years old.
I am a female.
I am a wife.
I am a daughter.
I am a sister.
I am a friend.
I am white-British.
I am a yoga teacher.
I am a writer.
I am a psychotherapist.
I am a harmonica player.
I am five-foot-one-and-a-half.

Take your list and sit or lay down somewhere comfortably, where you know you will not be disturbed. Take a few long, deep breaths and sink down into your heart centre. Read each sentence either aloud or silently to yourself, putting a long inhalation and exhalation between each word. For example, *'I (inhale, exhale) am (inhale, exhale) Nicole (inhale, exhale).'* Take a few long inhalations and exhalations before you move on to the next sentence. When you have worked your way through the whole list, simply repeat the words *'I am'* with a long inhalation and exhalation in between: *'I (inhale, exhale) am.'* Continue repeating *'I am'* in this way for a few minutes, or longer if you have the time. Eleven minutes, in accordance with the tradition of Kundalini yoga, is a good length of time for such a practice.

Allow the sense of *'I am'* to wash through you. Really feel into this sense of 'I'. Does it have a name, a gender, an ethnicity, a profession...? Or do the name, gender, colour, and profession arise within it and are witnessed by it? If thoughts wander off, gently bring them back with the breath and repetition of *'I am'*, allowing any resistance to be there without resisting it. Ask yourself, *'Who is the one being taken away by other thoughts?'* Return to the sense of who you are at the very deepest part of yourself. Sink into the knowledge that life is a journey from you back to you.

When the eleven minutes or so have passed, take a piece of paper and allow any thoughts or feelings to free-flow on to the page. This might come in the form of words, drawings etc. You might prefer to use clay, paints and so on. Or you might find yourself laying the paper to one side and dancing your expression out.

Finish by spending eleven minutes simply repeating the word 'I' with at least one inhalation and exhalation between each repetition. Again, feel into this sense of 'I'.

When we attempt to turn towards the sense of 'I', we may have the experience of being thrown back on ourselves. We may experience stillness, as opposed to anything with objective qualities. Our name is a 'thing' and we can turn towards our knowing of it. So, too, can we turn towards our knowing of our profession, our gender, and so on. Yet, we cannot turn towards the 'I', since it has no objective qualities. This 'I' is Awareness. It is Love. This 'I' is the one who is aware of the name of the person but is vaster than the name, the one who is aware of the body but expands beyond the body. Stay with this One and you may experience a sense of personal identity wavering or even dissolving. You may discover that you are none of the things you originally listed. You are the awareness of these things. You are the Awareness itself.

The body is a sticky aspect of 'I-am-ness'. So many of us have ascribed the 'I' to our physical body. Perhaps look over your list and highlight the aspects that pertain to your physical body; for example, your age, your gender, or your height. Then, notice how many of the other aspects are tied up with your body in some way. Given that we experience the physical world through our senses which, in turn, we experience through the body, each of the aspects we take ourselves to be are intrinsically entangled with the body at some level. Yet, as we explored in Chapter One, we came into this world without a sense that our identity is related to our body at all. Let us try another practice.

Mirror Gazing

Find a mirror (ideally a full-length mirror) and stand or seat yourself comfortably in front of it. Take time to settle into your position, using cushions or blankets to make yourself as cosy as possible. Notice any resistance to being in front of the mirror and stay with this resistance. Where do you feel the resistance in your body? Stay with the physical sensation of the resistance, without attaching any judgement to it. Feel into it, welcoming the resistance like a frightened child who requires your love and attention. If it helps, you can enlist the felt-sense of your allies—people and/or animals with whom you feel safe and from whom you have experienced support in the past. Solicit the sense of their support as you sit here.

When you are ready, close your eyes. Take a few moments to come to a place of stillness in your body, drawing your attention to your breath.

Notice your breath coming into, and going out of, your body. Notice your breath without judgement or trying to change anything about it. Stay with the awareness of your breath. Then, turn your attention to the one who is aware of your breath. Take your stand as the one who is observing and feeling your breath. Stay with this.

In your own time, open your eyes and meet your reflection in the mirror. Notice any changes in your breath and stay with these changes, without judgement or trying to change anything about them. Notice any other reactions to your reflection within your body and mind. Stay with these reactions without attempting to escape from them in any way.

Take a few moments to look into your own eyes. Breathe deeply, anchoring your breath in your heart centre, and, again, feel into any resistance. You might choose to stay with your eyes or you might like to turn your gaze to your whole face, your whole body, or a part of your body that you have a particularly hard time accepting. Notice where the seeing of your eyes, face, body, or body part arises. Notice that it arises in the same place or space as the awareness of your breath. Notice that it emerges in the same place as your awareness of the room in which you are sitting/standing. Witness how it arises in the same place as the hearing of any sounds in your environment.

Notice that there is a 'you' who looks at the reflection and a 'you' that you experience seeing. Which 'you' are you? Allow this question to resonate for a while, perhaps repeating it slowly to yourself with a deep inhalation and exhalation between each word:

'Which 'I' am I?'

'Am I the seer or the one who is seen?'

Move your eyes around the room and allow them to rest on whatever captures your attention. Notice how you do not identify with other objects in the same way in which you identify with your body. Yet, your awareness of these objects arises in the same place as your awareness of your body. Choose an object and look between this object and your reflection to check this out in your direct experience. Is the awareness of your reflection any different in quality than your awareness of other *objects? Or is there always a witnessing presence—a 'You'—that perceives everything in the same way?*

*Return your attention to the mirror. Try opening and closing your eyes. Where is the sense of your body experienced when you are looking at it? Where is it experienced when you are **not** looking at it? Check out, in your own experience, whether your awareness of your body arises in the same place in both instances.*

Maybe gaze upon a body part you dislike or have a hard time with. Perhaps you have told yourself it is too big, small, hairy, blemished, fat, or thin, or not muscular enough, or something like that. In your actual experience, can your knowing of this body part be separated from anything else that is known? In your experiencing of this body part, is there a line between your sense of this body part and the sense of the space in the room? Or between your experience of that body part and your experience of the sound of the birds singing? Or is your actual experience one of a seamless arising that is both nowhere and everywhere and belongs to no one?

Perhaps close your eyes again and direct your attention to the sensations in a disliked body part. Is there anything—aside from thought (whose job it is to separate)—in your direct experience that separates these sensations from any other(s)?

Take as much time as you need to explore the experience of perceiving your body. You might like to look directly at a part of your body, perhaps looking down at your legs or holding a hand directly in front of your eyes. Are you your hand or the one who perceives your hand? Are you your hand or are you the awareness of your hand: The Awareness itself?

We have been taught repeatedly that we are our body. However, when we return to our direct experience, we find that we are the one who is *aware* of the body, in the same way that we are the one who is aware of the room, tree, apple, and sunset. When we stay with our direct experience, we return to the sense we had as an infant—that the tree outside our nursery window was as close to us as our torso: Closer than close.

As we engage in this practice of taking our stand as the one who is aware of our body, we notice that our body has far less to do with 'us' than we had previously believed or understood. There appear to be three main stages that often unfold in this process:

1. *We believe our identities to be wrapped up in our physical body, including the appearance of our physical body.*
2. *We experience a separation between the one who is aware of our body and our body itself. Alongside this, there often emerges a sense that we are not our body at all, but, rather, are the one who is aware of our body.*
3. *We experience a remembering and a re-joining of our body and the awareness of our body. We experience ourselves as Awareness/Love and our body as a modulation of Awareness/ Love.*

This is not something that can be read to be understood. It requires direct experience. You need to check this out for yourself. Taking my word for it simply won't make the grade. If moving beyond your appearance-identity-focused pain is important to you, I implore you to make the practice of delving deeply into who you are your top priority. Ask yourself continually, in every moment available to you:

'Who am I?'
'Who am I at the deepest part of myself?'

Notice, ever more acutely, that the experience of your body comes and goes within your awareness. There are times in your life when you are not aware of your body at all. There are vast expanses of your body, in fact, which you are likely to be very rarely aware of. When was the last time, for example, that you were aware of the middle toe on your left foot? Your awareness of your body comes and goes, just as everything in your experience moves in and out of awareness. What is the only aspect of your experience that you never witness entering or departing? Notice that the only answer to this question is Awareness itself. It is possible to answer the question, *'Am I aware of my right kneecap?'* with a *'no'*. It is possible to answer the question, *'Am I aware of the size of my body?'* with a *'no'*. Yet, is it, or could it ever be, possible to answer in the negative to the question, *'Am I aware?'*

Rupert Spira describes this beautifully using the analogy of a television screen. The television screen is analogous to the open, empty space of awareness. While images colour the screen and capture the body-mind's attention, the screen itself remains unaffected and unaltered. The body is one such colour in the open space of awareness. We notice our body in the foreground, failing to pay attention to the screen in the background—the space of awareness on to which our body plays. The images on the screen are permeated with the screen, in the same way in which our body is permeated with awareness. The images are made of the screen. Our body is made of awareness, just as all objects in our experience are.

Every experience related to our body: Pain in our body, the seeing of our body, the feeling of sensations in our body, and so on—all arise within awareness. Could they arise outside of awareness? We have mistaken the finger for the moon it is pointing at. We have mistaken our body for who we are. When we return to our direct experience, we find that our body is no more or less Awareness than anything else, and is, therefore, no more or less 'us' than anything else.

When we really grasp this, any suffering attached to the physical appearance of our body drops away. Suffering can only be present when we have mistakenly wrapped our identity up in something we are not. When we take our stand as Awareness, the appearance of our body is no more painful to us than the appearance of the sunrise, since both are phenomena that arise in Awareness, and Awareness is who we are.

Societal myths—which most of the people around us will have taken on, to a greater or lesser extent—may continue to push against our new understanding. We may find ourselves oscillating for a while or may even sense ourselves being pulled back into the body-as-identity myth. Sometimes entirely. This was certainly my experience.

In one moment, I absolutely understood that I was the Love within which the body is witnessed. Then, a few weeks later, I would find tears springing to my eyes when I couldn't easily button up my jeans. They say that old habits die hard. It can be very difficult to maintain our stand as Awareness/Love when everyone around us is lamenting the extra pounds on their body, the blemishes on their skin, their lack of musculature, and so on. Many of us—particularly in the Western world—are bombarded with hundreds (if not thousands) of images expounding a certain body type on a daily basis. Our brains take these images on as being the body type that is needed to ensure our belongingness to the group, and, therefore, our survival. Thus, in the early stages, it often requires a moment-by-moment-vigilance and a moment-by-moment decision to maintain our stand as the witnessing presence as opposed to that which is being witnessed. Life, of course, is in the string of moments. It is in the details. Over time, our conditioning will update itself and less vigilance will be needed. For myself personally, the gap between a 'trigger' and remembering that I am the awareness of my body—not the body itself—is growing ever smaller. This remembrance is available to each of us, no matter how deeply entrenched in our struggles we have been or have become.

It can feel disheartening if—despite all our efforts and self-enquiry—we continue to agonise over the appearance of our body for a while. It may be that the appearance of our body goes out of focus for a time and then returns full-force—particularly during periods of body-change, such as pregnancy, illness, and ageing. As the body changes, its appearance may present itself to our awareness in a new wave. The invitation is to keep going! *'Keep up and you will be kept up,'* as Yogi Bhajan would often say. The invitation is one of commitment; to continuously remind ourselves of who we are and to continually retake our position as the loving, witnessing presence *as often as it takes, for as long as it takes.* As Yogi Bhajan reminded us, 'There *is actually no need to have a victory. You are the victory.'* Be the victory you are, however your efforts unfold. If this means refocusing your attention away from the appearance of the body to the one who is aware of the appearance of the body a thousand times a day, so be it. Tomorrow, it might be nine-hundred-and-ninety-nine times. If this seems tedious, notice that this supposition is resistance in a very clear form. Resistance is wonderful at disguising itself as boredom and the sense that something is a waste of time. This is not a waste of our time. This is the passport to our lived experience of the Freedom we already are.

The Seasons of the Changing Body

The appearance of our body changes throughout our lifetime. This is not a reality any of us can escape. We could describe our body as moving through various seasons. We are born into the spring of our body in early infancy—a time full of new life, possibility, supple limbs, growth, the gradual emergence from the ground (lying down to standing up), wonder, awe, and fresh discoveries. We continue to move through the spring during childhood, 'blossoming' into our adult bodies in adolescence and trying on different identities for size.

We then move into the summer of the life-cycle as our brain becomes fully-developed at around the age of twenty-five. This is a time for a greater exploration outside (of our family circle), developing careers, deepening romantic relationships, and perhaps starting a family of our own. Our body may feel more stable in its form at this time, although events such as pregnancy may alter the body in the most miraculous of ways.

As we come into middle-age, we move into the autumn of our lives. We perhaps begin to shed some of the demands we have historically placed on others and ourselves. We may begin to let go of the many social masks we have been wearing, feeling as though we no longer care so much about what people think of and say about us. We may begin to simplify our commitments. We may feel a deeper yearning to spend our time on meaningful, enriching pursuits. We may literally begin to shed the false self. Our body, at this stage, is beginning to age visibly. Grey hairs may emerge in ever greater numbers, as may wrinkles. Weight may increase or be shed. Height may reduce, and moisture is likely to be lost from the skin and hair.

As we enter old age, we come into the winter of our lives. Our body is often becoming colder, drier, smaller, and more crumpled. There may be a sense of hibernation and of a greater retreat from the social world. There is often a deepening sense of what is truly important and a further shedding of phenomena like social masks and social graces. The true Self is exposed, perhaps more than it has ever been in adult life. Illness and helplessness may ensue, prompting feelings of vulnerability. If support with self-care — like toileting, dressing, and feeding — is needed, it may feel as though we are returning to infancy. Thus, the seasons have come full-circle, as they always do. The body-mind is preparing for death, but Love is preparing for a new birth — for the next spring.

Of course, our springs, summers, autumns, and winters will not all look this way. Our bodies and our experiences are wonderfully unique, although the ageing process itself does, in some way, touch us all, if we live long enough. Welcoming and celebrating each season, as well as embracing all associated emotions with open arms, is the ongoing invitation to each of us. Welcoming the notion of the death of the body-mind is also a beautiful practice and nothing to be afraid of. You might like to try the following meditation as an example of this.

Deathbed Meditation

Lay down somewhere comfortably, perhaps on your bed or a yoga mat on the floor. Begin to deepen your breathing, taking full inhalations, as first your abdomen, then your chest, then your clavicle area expands. Exhale completely, allowing first your clavicle, then your chest area, and lastly, your abdomen, to drop back towards the spine. Allow each part of your body to relax as fully as possible, perhaps starting by relaxing each toe in turn, then moving through your feet, ankles, calves, knees, thighs, hips, and torso, and continuing to loosen all the muscles in your body, all the way up to the crown of your head.

As you lay here, imagine that you are lying on your deathbed and these are the last few moments of your life. You might like to visualise who is there with you, or perhaps you are alone.

Notice the emotions this visualisation brings up for you. Feel into them fully. If you notice any resistance or fear, welcome these also with a loving, accepting embrace.

You might find your mind passing over the significant events in your life. You might find that specific people come to mind. Allow whatever comes up to come up. There is no right or wrong here.

Take a deep inhalation, imagining your breath going all the way down to the base of your spine. Breathe out fully and lightly suspend your breath. For a few seconds or so, while your breath is suspended on the exhale, sense that the body-mind has died. Sink into your awareness of this. Notice that your awareness continues, and that it remains untouched by the death of the body-mind. Notice that death is something which occurs within your awareness.

When you are ready, take a deep inhalation, allowing any emotions and reactions to these emotions to emerge unbidden. Take some time with these emotions. You might like to give your body a hug, take a walk in nature, or connect with someone you love. You may notice how vibrant the world seems to be after having 'come back from death'.

Drink this in, but also allow experiences which are unlike this, such as residual fear, doubt, and pain, to surface and to be felt. Whatever is happening is what is happening. All is well.

Either before or after this meditation, you might like to ask yourself the following questions:

- *Who do I most admire? Why? What legacy did/will they leave the world after their body-mind died/dies? Can I recognise parts of myself in them? (We tend to admire people who carry/emit disowned, true Self aspects of our beingness.)*
- *If I had three months left to live, what would I be doing today? Tomorrow? For the next three months? On what and with whom would I desire to focus my attention?*
- *If I had three months left to live, how would I feel about the appearance of my body?*
- *How would I most like to be remembered? After my body-mind has died, would I like people to remember me for the way I looked or for the things I did and the way I made people feel?*
- *What message would my dead body-mind want to give to my alive body-mind? How can I take up this message in this moment? Today? For the rest of the life my body-mind spends on Earth?*

Epilogue

Much of the population does not look at their bodies and see Love shining back at them. Many people see primarily a mass of judgements made about their body in the past. It is very powerful to stand in front of a mirror and commit to really seeing our bodies, in the present moment, perhaps for the very first time. Not our thoughts and judgements about our bodies, but our bodies themselves.

I remember the first time I stood in front of a mirror with the specific intention of really seeing my body, as opposed to seeing the past. I set my intention: *I see my body in **this** moment.* I looked. I still saw 'too much' staring back at me—a mass of things I would like to change, a physicality I could hardly identify with and found very difficult to accept. So again, I uttered, *'I see my body in **this** moment.'* I allowed myself to be open to dropping past ideas—ideas I had previously clung to as though they were as vital to life as breathing. I allowed myself to come to the mirror *'without memory or desire,'* as Bion so poignantly put it. I allowed the inner dialogue of my mind to wash over me without attaching any meaning, truth, or identity to it.

I gazed at my body in the present moment and momentarily saw a matrix of energy where my body was standing—clever and beautiful little cells dancing around a life-force that kept my heart beating and the body alive. It was as though I was seeing a body made up of tiny sparks of light, a body utterly intelligent and awesome in design. I began to cry. My body was not my flesh and had nothing to do with how many inches of fat sat on my bones. My body was a miraculous and divine clothing for an Aliveness, a Beingness that cared nothing for appearances. And in that moment, I saw reality as it really is.

Consider how your body came into the world. The cell that began your physical body was so tiny that you could fit a million of them on to the head of a pin. Within this cell was everything you would ever need. Written within this tiny cell was your eye colour, hair colour, and how rapidly your skin would shed and regrow. From this cell came everything that you physically are. As an acorn holds the entire oak tree, this cell held the entirety of you as a physical entity on this planet. Yet, everything from that point onwards was beyond the remit of that cell. That cell did not create other cells, creating and creating until you had a body. Cells do not create other cells. Something beyond the measurement of physics was going on, something physicists can't see under a microscope or explain with laws or theories. It is, physicists say, almost as if there is a 'mind' behind these cells, orchestrating them and thinking them into being.

Something beyond physical matter is creating and playing. When scientists try to look for this orchestrator, this cosmic playwright, they come away perplexed and empty-handed. When we ourselves look for this life-force driving our experience, we, too, come away wanting. We find only thoughts, perceptions, and sensations arising and dissolving. The place they emerge from and fall back into is a total mystery. It is absolute emptiness and utter fullness tangentially.

This 'one that cannot be found', this emptiness, and this aliveness is our pure essence. We could also call it Love. Love encompasses all seeming things, while everything else in our experience exists in polarities. This body versus that body, black versus white, pain versus pleasure, and so on. Thoughts also exist in polarities. Therefore, it is not possible to have a truly neutral thought. We do not see neutral bodies since our thoughts about bodies are not neutral. They are, in fact, laden with judgements. These judgements may revolve around food and weight and may also be linked to the purpose, strength, meaning, and symbolism of our bodies. When we pin our sense of identity on the appearance of our physical body, the body becomes decidedly biased. It can literally become our biggest battleground.

The thoughts about the appearance of our bodies are only thoughts. They are not reality. Even those seemingly pure thoughts—the holy thoughts, the compassionate thoughts, and the Oneness thoughts—they are still only thoughts. Concepts are not truth. Concepts are only ever concepts.

I could take a weighing scale out now and step on it. I could look at the number—this abstraction that somehow gets interpreted with meaning by thought—and have any number of reactions: Indifference, surprise, elation, depression, terror, or joy. The reaction I have to that number will be totally different to the reaction another person of the same height and build as myself. So, the pain, of course, is not in the number or in the concept in any way. The pain is in the meaning we make of the number. Yet, we rarely stop to consider where the meanings constructed by thoughts have come from.

When I understood that I am Love expressing itself in a physical form, the number on the scale ceased to mean anything to me. Love has no weight; thus, I have no weight. I am weightless and utterly free.

Just as the infant's earliest months are outside of cognition, so, too, is the experience of freedom. The most expansive experiences we can have as body-minds are totally outside of thought and thinking.

Thinking cannot exist in the present moment. It is always one step behind. We have an experience and then thought arises. It is always 'too late'. Thought and the present moment always have distance between them. Thought is only ever in the business of catch-up and commentary. What is the experience of Existence without the commentary? We do not have to wonder because we all know this. We have all had moments where time seemed to stand still, moments—or, rather, non-moments—within which our thoughts and the notion of a separate body-mind were totally suspended.

The experience of feeling uncomfortable in our body is also always outside the present moment. Our thoughts assert that, right now, we are feeling fat, puny, ugly, spotty, or whatever it is. If we return to our actual experience, we find that this is never the case. Rather, we have a sensation and our thoughts come in afterwards to label it as the feeling of being too fat, ugly, blemished, or whatever it is. However, in the moment of the feeling—the moment within which the sensation arises—there is only sensation arising. As infants, there was only sensation arising without our thoughts calling it this thing or that thing. In animals, it seems to be this way. Pure experiencing. This pure experiencing of the body without thought has no interest in labelling of any kind. Sensation itself does not label sensation.

It is the nature of some forms to be one way, and other forms to be another. It is the nature of the rose to look like the rose, and the nature of the daisy to look like the daisy. It is the nature of one rose to have many petals, and the nature of another to have fewer. It is the nature for one rose to have many thorns, and the other to have fewer. Does one rose look at another rose and agonise, *'Why has that rose got less petals than me?'* That sounds ridiculous, doesn't it? Yet, we somehow look at other body-forms and compare this form to that form. *'Why does he have a flatter stomach than me? Why does she have less facial hair than me?'* It pains us because we have decided that certain body-forms are good and others are bad. We suffer because we believe we can become more lovable by altering how we look.

Our conditioning ignites thoughts that this kind of a body is good, and this kind of a body is bad. We do not agonise over the size of our feet, for example—or very rarely so—because we have not been told this has something to do with our lovability. It all comes back—as, indeed, everything does—to love.

We are not our bodies. Yet, we are called to honour our bodies as the beautiful temples they are. I have learned to be eternally grateful for each part of my body. Each facet of our physicality has a wonderful and important job to do, and each of these parts needs energy to do it. Now, when I look at my legs in the mirror, I thank them for holding me up and moving me to where I would like to go instead of crying about how broad they are. I thank them for being strong, for not buckling beneath me, and for bending at the knee to allow me to sit down when I am weary. Sometimes, when I look at my body in the mirror, I imagine what it will look like after the soul leaves it. One day, this body will die and begin to disintegrate. The fat, muscles, and tendons in my legs will be gone, leaving only bone behind.

As children, we were often told that we needed to be the 'best'. To be the 'best' at thinness, you need to become dreadfully thin. If you are living out this story of trying to be the best at being thin, you will suffer when you see somebody who is thinner— whether objectively or subjectively—than you are. Of course, there will always be someone who is thinner, has clearer skin, is more muscular, has less body hair, and so on. It is not possible to become the 'best' or the thinnest (or whatever else you are pinning your hope on to), but it *is* possible to move beyond the notions that you need to be this-or-that to be worthy of love and attention. The purpose of life is to be who we truly are, which is Love itself. It is no more complex than this. If we are who we truly are without reserve, the whole point of life is accomplished. So simple. So beautiful.

People's behaviour towards us may completely change when we stop dieting, going to the gym, covering up our blemishes, or whatever else it might be. On the surface of things, this might seem difficult at first. Our thoughts may suggest that we are getting less attention, and this may be confused—again, by our thoughts—with the notion that we are getting less love. Yet, love is not linked to attention; at least, not in the way most of us have conceptualised it. Love simply *is*. It is not given, nor can it be taken away. It does not move from one person to another person. Love happens when the identity embedded in the body-mind—

the sense of separation—drops away.

The attention we get as human beings from other human beings is ninety-nine per cent attention for a pseudo-self. Most of it is wrapped up in games. *I'll play the part of Nicole who is always mild and eager to please and you play along with that, okay? And I'll play along with your character, who is cheerful and good-humoured. I'll bring my conceptualisation of you to each of our meetings and you'll bring your conceptualisation of me. Then, we'll give each other what we think we want and need and everything will be okay. Okay?*

When do we truly meet another without the games, past conceptualisations, and suppositions? Can we ever truly meet another while there is any semblance of separation between us?

The thoughts linked to appearance-focused identity struggles are fear-based. Some say that fear is the opposite of love, but I am not sold on this one. If everything is love, then surely, fear is an aspect of love also. Therefore, there is a fearlessness implicit in the fear. There is nothing more liberating than looking fear in the face and diving completely into trust. Into Love.

Our fear may seem to be based in a dysfunctional family, a volatile early attachment relationship, a terrifying sense of unsafety, a feeling of being unloved, a desire for thinness, a perfectionist nature turned in on the wrong focus... Are these the reasons we struggle? Yes and no. But mostly, no. These struggles are bigger than the self, vaster than other singular people, and broader than the family. This wider breeding ground is embedded in the 'fight-and-resist' mentality of our modern age. Its antidote is to surrender. As Yogi Bhajan explained, *'Our only power is our power to be powerless.'* At some point, we come to understand that we are being invited to surrender in the fight against who we are.

Freefalling into pure beingness is a terrifying and beautiful experience. It is utterly transformative. Looking in the mirror from this place is a prayer; a conscious expression of Love. When I look into the mirror these days, I regularly see something of unexpected magnificence. Often, something will catch my attention, like my eyes, and I will find myself marvelling at the myriad of colours and their impossibly intricate pattern. Or perhaps I will notice my belly and gawp in wonder at how it expands with each inhalation without anything deciding that. Sometimes, I'll catch myself become enraptured by the pattern of creases on my knuckle or the paleness of the small scar beneath my left wrist. I can become lost in my body in the same way I can become lost in a beautiful morning sky or a bird in flight. It is all so mysterious, this life that is happening and this being-ness that is being. Object and subject dissolve in these moments—the body and the One who is aware of the body are One Beingness, One Love.

The truth is that there is no good or bad, right or wrong, up or down, pure or impure. Eating a pear is love expressing itself in the same way that eating a slice of cake—or whatever food the person does or does not attach guilt and shame to—is love expressing itself. Eat the cake or do not eat the cake. It does not matter. All is exactly as it can only be.

The invitation here is to utterly surrender to everything as it is: Your body, your thoughts, your emotions... everything! This is simple and, yet, totally earthshattering. No need to work anything out. There is nothing to be worked out, and thoughts cannot 'get' this anyway. Simply welcome and feel whatever arises. Make friends with your emotions. Allow everything to emerge and to be exactly as it is.

There are moments when the sense of separation—the sense of yourself as a separate body-mind—dissolves and you experience just awareness and raw aliveness. The yogis call this *Samadhi*. Perhaps it happens when you are absorbed in gardening, when you are watching a child play, or when you walk in nature. It also seems to happen in the gaps between thoughts. It also happens in deep sleep. The personal you 'disappears'.

What is being spoken about here is no different to that. We

have the experience every day when we fall asleep or daydream. Then, we 'wake up' and slip back into the story of a separate 'me' being a body-mind, making choices and steering a life along.

We drop our hatred of our body when we stop seeking freedom from our hatred. As Yogi Bhajan reminded us, 'Do *not seek. See.'* When everything is permitted to be exactly as it is and our emotions are truly felt, wholeness is experienced everywhere: In the reflection in the mirror, the number on the scale, the tightness or looseness of our jeans, and the curve of our hips. Everywhere!

As the sense of identity related to the body-mind dissolves, so, too, does the fear of death, being unlovable, being rejected, being too fat, and not being good enough... all gone. Because there is no one to die and no one to be rejected. The lover leaving you, the lover staying with you, the person calling you beautiful, the person calling you ugly, the pain in the centre of your chest, and the lightness in the centre of your chest—are all Love expressing itself. We have convinced ourselves somehow that this thing is good, and the other is bad. We have split up everything according to polarities, or points along a trajectory of polarity. Our thoughts can only comprehend a polarised world. So, our thoughts will come in with a 'but' as soon as we say that the acne is love expressing itself in equal measure to the sunrise. Yet, it is so, and has always been.

All our searches are freedom projects. Yet, freedom has never left us. Freedom is who we are.

That freedom doesn't come from anything or anywhere. It is everything and nothing. It *is*. Trying to find it is *like the eye trying to see itself or the tooth trying to bite itself*, as the yogis put it. It is like a fish looking for water. It is *immersed* in the water. If we put our hands over our eyes, we cannot see our hands; yet, *all* we can see is our hands! Freedom is closer than close. The moment we suppose that we are a body-mind seeking freedom is the moment this reality is veiled.

We are already free and have always been free. This includes freedom from our compulsions and our fears. It might not feel like this after we have polished off yet another full packet of biscuits and find ourselves steeped in shame, but we are! There is an open, aware presence that witnessed the act and is totally untouched by it. This open, aware presence couldn't care less if you ate the biscuits, since it cannot be altered by anything, and yet, pervades everything. *This* is who you are. When you experience this, behaviours that do not serve you will drop away *naturally*. You will not need to hide the packet of biscuits from yourself. You will fully feel the feelings you are trying to escape or soothe by eating that whole packet of biscuits and then you will no longer have any need to consume them all. You might enjoy a couple because you are hungry or fancy a tasty bite. But you will not feel controlled by them.

At this point, some of the earlier practices that might have helped you—like having a meal plan, covering up the mirrors in the house, refraining from buying binge foods, and so on— will no longer be needed. You could have a whole house full of weighing scales and not feel compelled to step on a single one of them. You will know, with every fibre of your being, that:

Losing weight is not going to change who you are.
Having clear skin is not going to change who you are.
Getting cosmetic surgery on your nose is not going to change who you are.

You know that you are Love and that Love has no weight, height, shape, need of starvation, or need of bingeing... no need of anything at all. It is totally self-satisfied in every moment, for no reason at all. It is perpetually saturated in causeless joy. This causeless joy is there in every moment of your life, however covered up it might seem.

These are not possibilities for ten years' time, next year, next month, or even tomorrow. This is a possibility *now* and is *always and only now* a possibility. Notice this *now*. Take a breath and take your stand as the one who is aware of your body but is not your body. Take your stand as Love. Notice how your body is something that arises in your awareness — an Awareness that remains unchanged by *anything*, including any alteration to your body. Know this and you will know who you are.

Answer the question 'Who am I?' and all other questions will drop away. Life will flow effortlessly as, indeed, it always has been—you simply didn't notice as you tried to push it in this or that direction. Find out who you are as though your life depended on it. Yet, also know that all is well, whatever you do and whichever way you look at it.

Appendix One

Connecting with and Supporting Others Who Are Struggling

Given the law of averages, we probably all know someone who is experiencing food and body image issues to varying degrees. It can be agonising to watch somebody we care about deny themselves adequate nutrition, overeat their body into a state of physical danger, or shed tears over the size of their hips or nose, when to us, they look 'just fine'.

There can be a strong drive to reassure the person, offer solutions, and try and 'fix' them and their suffering in some way. This typically comes from good intentions and a place of love. Yet, it is unlikely to be the most effective way of offering our support.

As we have explored together, food and body image struggles are a body-based experience, the roots of which tend to live in our implicit, procedural memory and in the right side of our brain. Therefore, to connect with the person we are trying to support, we are invited to meet them through our body, emotions, and the right side of our brains—as opposed to the left side, with its remit of logic, language, linear thinking, and problem solving.

The first step is to acknowledge the emotional experience in the other person's body through our own body. The right side of our brain is less concerned with the words we use than with direct, sensory-based experiences. Our tone of voice, eye contact, facial expression, posture, prosody, gesture, and energy, as neuropsychiatrist Dan Siegel reminds us, are the language of the right brain and of the primitive brain also. They are also the primary language we used to attune to our primary caregivers as infants, of course.

We acknowledge the emotional experience of the other person

by feeling the emotion in our own body. As we have explored, the core emotion underlying food and body struggles is the fundamental fear of being unloved. Can we connect to this fear inside ourselves? Can we really feel into it? As we do so, can we maintain respectful eye contact, a soft facial expression, an open posture, and a compassionate tone of voice?

The right brain experiences and responds through the senses. Therefore, we can connect right brain to right brain, by employing the senses, such as through the timbre and pitch of our voice, our proximity, our use of touch, and so on. Laying a hand on the other's shoulder or offering them a hug (if touch feels safe and good for them) before launching into any kind of dialogue can allow for a deep connection to take place. This enables the person to feel witnessed, heard, understood, attuned to, contained, validated, and, therefore, loved—the very feelings their behaviours are seeking in the first place.

The call, then, is to respond to the underlying emotions, as opposed to jumping straight into interacting with and addressing the behaviours. This can be tricky to do if the person themselves is trying to draw you into a reassurance-based conversation; for example, a conversation about how much they ought to eat for dinner or whether their hips look big in the pair of trousers they are wearing. Such a conversation might be gently redirected towards a right-brain-to-right-brain exchange in the following way:

Joe: 'I can't stop thinking about how puny I look. I keep going to the gym, but my muscles never seem to get any bigger. It makes me want to stay at home and hide away all day. I can't face people. I really hate myself.'

You: (in a soft even tone, leaning towards Joe, feeling into the emotional responses in your body) 'I am so sorry you feel like that, Joe. That sounds like a scary place to be in. I can feel how hard it is for you to face people. I feel really moved to give you a hug right now. Can I?'

(Embrace.)

Joe: 'I just don't know what to do anymore. I'm exhausted by spending all my spare time at the gym. Nothing seems to make me feel better about myself.'

You: 'It must be really hard to feel so exhausted. It all sounds like so much effort, and so draining. I can feel a sense of hopelessness in my body when you talk about it. Is that how it feels for you?'

Joe: 'Yes. It feels utterly hopeless.' (Begins to cry.)

(Touch Joe's shoulder firmly and reassuringly.)

You: 'I'm wondering what that sense of hopelessness is like for you, Joe.'

Joe: 'It feels like there is no future for me unless I can make my body more attractive, so I may as well not bother anymore.'

You: 'You feel like not bothering anymore?'

Joe: 'Well, what's the point? Nothing changes. I am puny, and I'll always be puny. I'll never have a girlfriend and I'll be alone for the rest of my life. It's hopeless.'

You: 'It sounds like you have a real fear of being alone, Joe.'

Joe: 'Doesn't everyone?'

You: 'I am not so interested in everyone else right now. I'm interested in you.'

Joe: 'I hate the thought of being all alone. It terrifies me.'

You: 'It must be tough to be so terrified of being alone. It makes me feel cold in my chest when you talk about it.'

Joe: 'Yes. It's a cold, icy feeling. I cannot bear it.'

You: (begin to move into the left brain) 'I wonder what would help you bear it, Joe. I wonder if getting bigger muscles is really the answer or whether it might go deeper than that...'

Joe: 'I know, I know. Part of me knows that going to the gym isn't going to fix how I feel. But I need to do something. I can't just spend the rest of my life all alone without trying to make it easier for other people to love me.'

You: 'You think that other people do not find it easy to love you?'

Joe: 'I don't think they do.'

You: 'I am sorry you feel like that, Joe. Please tell me more about this sense that people do not find it easy to love you.'

And so, the conversation would continue. The point is that it would have been very easy to jump straight into telling Joe he doesn't look puny and doesn't need to keep going to the gym, but this would have been your left brain trying to connect with Joe's right brain, which simply does not work. Joe would not have had the experience of being validated (and wouldn't have believed your reassurances anyway); thus, potentially pushing him further into a sense of separation and shame.

In addition to the way we respond to our loved ones in the moment, the greatest and most transformational gift we can offer them is to delve into and assimilate our own emotions, whatever they might be. This is even more pertinent if we are parenting someone with food and body image issues, but it is important for friends and other family members also. Not only will the clearing and integrating of our own emotional experiences provide a space in which we can attune to, connect with and support the emotional experience of our loved ones, but it will also provide a personal template we can draw upon as we walk our loved one through the process. For these reasons, it is my very firm belief that any treatment for food and body struggles absolutely must include and encompass those who are in closest relationship with the person who is struggling. Food and body image struggles both emerge and heal in the context of relationships. Often, the person is the 'symptom carrier' for the whole family or subsystem. Therefore, the whole family or subsystem requires healing, not solely the person themselves.

All the struggles we engage in as human beings are, at their root, the struggle to feel lovable and to be loved. As *A Course In Miracles* teaches us, *'Everything is an act of love or a call for love.'* Healing naturally occurs in the context of this love. Our love, therefore, is the most profound and transformative gift we can offer someone who is agonising over food and/or their body. All the conversations, meal plans, reassurances, logic, food parcels, and books will not get us there (although, they can certainly be helpful at stages along the journey). Love will get us there. If we can support someone not only with our love but also by helping them to remember that they *are* Love, we have provided a tremendous service to that human being. Their lives will never again be the same, and neither will our own.

Yogi Bhajan explained that, *'Our presence is our purity.'* We can be a source of healing for others by our very presence. It is less about what we say or the actions we take. It has much more to do with how we connect heart-to-heart in each moment. It has much more to do with who we are.

The Story of the Candle That Wanted to Be Lit

A young, little candle heard that there would be an international congress for candles in a cave somewhere in India. The little candle was very excited. The title of the congress was, 'How to Become Lit'. The little candle had wanted to learn how to become lit for many years; for, since his birth, he had always been in darkness.

And so, the little candle travelled for many miles and came to a dark, dark cave in India. Already, thousands of candles were there. For the next few days, the little candle listened to the older candles talk about how to become lit. The little candle took extensive notes. He wanted to become lit more than anything else in the world.

After four days of lectures, the little candle began to become disheartened. Surely, becoming lit wasn't as complicated as this. For all these hours, he had been only listening in the darkness. The little candle wanted some action! Feeling despondent, he stepped outside the cave and stood beneath the stars.

'Please!' the little candle called out to the universe. 'I feel lost and I do not know what to do. Please show me the way to become lit.' As he stood there, the little candle saw a small light flickering in the distance. Intrigued, the little candle felt compelled to follow the light

to its source.

The little candle walked for what felt like many miles. As he got closer, he realised that the light was, indeed, a lit candle! His excitement could barely be contained.

Upon reaching the beautiful, flickering candle, the little candle was almost too awestruck to speak. Finally, he mustered enough courage and called out desperately to the lit candle.

'Please,' he said. 'For so many years, I have been searching for a way to become lit. For the last four days, I have been attending a conference about this very thing, and yet, I am still in darkness. I would be unspeakably grateful if you could please tell me how to become lit, just like you.'

The older candle smiled at his new little friend. 'You want to know how to become lit?' he asked playfully. 'It is easy. I used to be like you. Wandering around, looking for someone to tell me how to light myself up. Then I learnt that it is so very easy. Look. All you need to do is to come close to me and allow yourself to touch me. Then, you will find that you will become lit without any effort on either of our parts.' 'Really?' gasped the little candle in amazement. 'Can it really be that simple?' 'Sure,' replied the lit candle. 'Come. Touch me and see just how easy it is.' So, the little candle came closer to the lit candle and touched him. Suddenly, he was alight! 'Wow!' he exclaimed. 'That is really beautiful! Please come back to the cave with me and show all the candles there how they, too, can become lit like us.' 'There is no need for me to come,' responded the bigger candle. 'Just go to that cave, allow the other candles to be touched by you, and they, too, will become lit.' So, the little candle returned to the cave… you can imagine how the story ends.

Appendix Two

Contributing/Engaging in Acts of Service

We discover what we have by giving it away. We discover who we are by giving ourselves away.

It is important not to confuse the act of giving ourselves away with the act of fawning. Fawning is one corner of the 'fight, flight, freeze, or fawn' square. To fawn is to lay aside our own needs and act servilely towards another to keep them close, keep ourselves safe, and survive.

Sharing the love that we are is a different act entirely. It comes from a place of abundance, as opposed to a place of destitution. As the tree, so Jesuit priest Anthony de Mello teaches us, offers its shade to whoever comes under its branches, offering its very 'tree-ness' totally freely and completely indiscriminately, so we offer our love, our very being-ness to everyone who might pass by, totally freely and completely indiscriminately. Show me the tree that called the traveller back for some water because it offered its shade. There is no trade for the tree, the flower, the sand, or the ocean, and there is no trade for us. *Give me your love and I'll give you mine...* This is not the language of the heart.

We are all serving something. Literally anything can become our altar; whether we are serving other people, food, exercise, cosmetic surgery... what we choose to give our energy and attention to is that which we serve. Though it can be challenging, try to discover which words you tend to use most often both in your own thoughts and in your verbalisations with others. These words are your *Jappa*, meaning that which you repeat continuously, your mantra if you will. These words represent that which you worship. They point to where your altar is. When we take our stand as Love, we naturally transform the language we use and the altar at which we serve. We organically come into

193

the service of others. This service amplifies our experience of being Love and having love. We create a virtuous cycle. We heal and are healed in the most multidimensional ways.

Therefore, finding ways to serve our families and our communities tends to be an organic part of the process of moving beyond appearance-focused identity struggles. Some ideas include:

- Inviting neighbours/friends/people in your community to your house for a simple meal, poetry reading, drawing session, sharing circle, yoga etc.
- Going to the house of a community member/friend etc. and cooking them a meal, cleaning their house, helping them with the weeding etc.
- Volunteering at local residential homes for the elderly, children's centres, animal rescue centres, charitable organisations, homeless shelters, food banks, or community allotments.
- Starting a community project like dog walking for the housebound, baking cakes and delivering them to your elderly neighbours, clothes-swap initiatives for the less fortunate, or community planting projects.
- Connecting to others through your creative gifts, such as by running workshops for poetry, painting, creative writing, or sewing, thereby using your creative pursuits as a platform to share your experiences and extend support to others with similar experiences.
- Lobbying for causes that are close to your heart.
- Offering random acts of kindness to your community, such as posting an inspirational book to five neighbours, spending an afternoon picking up litter, leaving a bunch of flowers on a random car with a note of kindness, offering a blanket and some homemade soup to a homeless person, bringing a receptionist a cup of coffee, or making two

lunch boxes and giving one away.
- ... and at least a million other possibilities!

Serving others may also support us in the earlier stages of our struggles. This was certainly the case for me. I began volunteering at a residential home for the elderly when I came out of a lengthy hospitalisation under the diagnosis of anorexia. I was still rather emotionally shaky at the time, trying desperately to keep my head above water, while feeling the same intense hatred for myself that I had already felt for many years. I remember travelling on the train to that residential home and repeating to myself silently all the way, *I may be a monster, but at least I can make Norah a cup of tea.* What kept me going was the notion that no matter how ugly and unlovable I was, I could still do some good in this world and bring some kindness into the life of another person. It gave me a purpose and a reason to pull myself out of bed and away from the mirror each morning. It gave me hope.

As I have learned that I am a good and loving human being over the years, my experience of service has changed entirely. I no longer hang on to this service as a reason for living. Instead, it flows naturally and joyfully, and thus, the connection I have with others is more spacious and much deeper. However, I do not regret those years in the residential home and I know that people like Norah were glad I went along. So, we can serve at any stage; initially, perhaps, to have an experience of ourselves as Love, and later, to give ourselves as the Love we know we are.

Appendix Three

Selected Kundalini Chants for Healing

Kundalini chants or mantras are typically in Gurmukhi, a sacred Indian language, and occasionally, in English. These mantras contain the vibrations of peace, connection, and many other qualities. They are understood by their impact, even if the meaning of each word is not known. Knowing the meaning of the words, however, adds another layer of effectiveness. You can find many more chants on the Spirit Voyage Mantropedia, located at: www.spiritvoyage.com/mantrahome.aspx. You can also access Celestial Communications recorded by myself at www.youtube.com/c/PointofLight. Celestial Communications are, in the tradition of Kundalini Yoga, moving meditations; mantras with accompanying movements.

Adi Mantra (for tuning in and connecting to Love)
Ong Namo Guru Dev Namo
I bow to the Creative Wisdom; I bow to the Divine Teacher within.

Mangala Charn Mantra (for connecting to a sense of safety and containment)
Aad Guray Nameh Jugaad Guray Nameh Sat Guray Nameh Siri
Guru Dayvay Nameh

Ajai Alai (to lift one from depression and anger)
Ajai Alai Abhai Abai Abhoo Ajoo Anaas Akaas Aganj Abhanj
Alakkh Abhakkh Akaal Dyaal Alaykh Abhaykh Anaam
Akaam Agaaha Adhaaha Anaathay Pramaathay Ajonee
Amonee Na Raagay Na Rangay Na Roopay Na Raykhay
Akarmang Abharmang Aganjay Alaykhay
Invincible, Indestructible.

Fearless, Unchanging.
Unformed, Unborn.
Imperishable, Etheric.
Unbreakable, Impenetrable.
Unseen, Unaffected.
Undying, Merciful.
Indescribable, Un-costumed.
Nameless, Desire-less.
Unfathomable, Incorruptible.
Unmastered, Destroyer.
Beyond birth, Beyond silence.
Beyond love, Beyond colour.
Beyond form, Beyond shape.
Beyond karma, Beyond doubt.
Unconquerable, Indescribable.
(Lovely recordings—Ajeet Kaur, Mirabai Ceiba)

Chattra Chakkra Vartee (for releasing fear)
Chattra Chakkra Vartee,
Chattra Chakkra Bhugatay,
Suyambhav Subhang Sarab Daa Saraab Jugatay.
Dukaalan Pranasee, Diaalang Saroopay,
Sadaa Ang Sangay, Abhangang Bibhutaay.
You are pervading in all the four directions, the Enjoyer in all the
four directions. You are self-illuminated, profoundly beautiful,
and united with all. Destroyer of the torments of birth and death,
embodiment of mercy, you are ever within us. You are the everlasting
giver of indestructible power.
(Lovely recordings—Nirinjan Kaur, Satwant Kaur, Snatam
Kaur)

Mul Mantra (the root mantra from which a spiritual
foundation is built)
Ek ong kaar, sat naam, karataa purakh, nirbho, nirvair

Akaal moorat, ajoonee, saibhang, gur prasaad. Jap!
Aad such, jugaad such, Hai bhee such, Naanak hosee bhee
such.

One Creator. Truth is His name. Doer of everything. Fearless,
Revenge-less, Undying, Unborn, Self-Illuminated, The Guru's gift,
Meditate! True in the beginning. True through all the ages. True
even now. Oh, Nanak, it is forever true.

(Lovely recordings—Satwant Kaur, Snatam Kaur)

Re Man (or Ray Man) Shabad (for wisdom and purity)
Ray man eh bidh jog kamao
Singhee saach akapat kanthala
Dhiaan bibhoot charhaao
Taatee gaho aatam bas kar kee
Bichaa naam adhaarang
Baaje param taar tat har ko
Upajay raag rasaarang
Ughatay taan tarang rang atay giaan geet bandhaanang
Chak rahay dayv daanav mun
Chhak chaak biyom bivaanang
Aatam upadays bhays sanjam ko
Jaap so ajapa jaapay
Sada rahay kanchan si kaya
Kaal na kabahoo byaapay
Oh, my mind, practise Yoga in this way:
Let Truth be your horn, sincerity your necklace, and meditation the
ashes you apply on your body.
Catch your burning soul (self) and stop the flames. Let the soul (self)
be the alms bowl in which you collect the sweet Naam and this will be
the only support you will ever need.
The Universe plays its divine music. The sound of reality is shrill,
but this is where God is.
When you listen to the reality from this place of awareness, the sweet
essence of Raag arises.

Waves of melodies, emotions, and passions arise and flow through
you. Bind yourself with the song of God.
The Universe spins like a potter's wheel and from it fly demons and
angels. The sage listens to this and instead of getting caught in either
one, the sage drinks in the nectar of the heavens and is carried to the
heavens in a divine chariot.
Instruct and clothe yourself in self-control. Meditate unto infinity
until you are meditating without meditating.
In this way, your body shall remain forever golden, and death shall
never approach you.
(Lovely recordings—Ajeet Kaur, Snatam Kaur)

Sat Nam
Truth is my Identity.

Further Reading List

Psychoanalytic Thought

Bion, WR (1994). *Learning from Experience*. Jason Aronson, Incorporated.

Freud, S. & Strachey, JE (1964). *The Standard Edition of the Complete Psychological Works of Sigmund Freud*.

Klein, M. (1997). *Envy and Gratitude: And Other Works, 1946–1963*. Random House.

Klein, M. (1997). *The Psycho-Analysis of Children*. Random House.

Klein, M. (2002). *Love, Guilt and Reparation: and other works 1921–1945* (Vol. 1). Simon and Schuster.

Mahler, MS (1968). *On Human Symbiosis and the Vicissitudes of Individuation. Infantile Psychosis, Volume 1*.

Symington, J. (1996). *The Critical Thinking of Wilfred Bion*. Routledge.

Winnicott, DW (1965). 1960 Ego distortion in Terms of True and False Self. *The Maturational Processes and the Facilitating Environment*.

Winnicott, DW (1971). *Playing and Reality*. Psychology Press.

Nutrition and Gut Health

Collen, A. (2016). *10% Human: How Your Body's Microbes Hold the Key to Health and Happiness*. William Collins.

Enders, G. (2017). *Gut: New Revised Expanded Edition*. Scribe UK.

Leggett, D. (2014). *Helping Ourselves: A Guide to Traditional Chinese Food Energetics*. Meridian Press.

Mayer, E. (2016). *The Mind-Gut Connection: How the Hidden Conversation Within Our Bodies Impacts Our Mood, Our Choices, and Our Overall Health*. Harper Wave.

Reichstein, G. (1999). *Wood Becomes Water: Chinese Medicine in Everyday Life*. Kodansha American Inc.

Tiwari, M. (1994). *Ayurveda: A Life of Balance: The Complete Guide to Ayurvedic Nutrition and Body Types with Recipes.* Healing Arts Press.

Meditation, Kundalini and Non-Duality

Bhajan, Y. & Khalsa, GS (1998). *The Mind: Its Projections and Multiple Facets.* Kundalini Research Institute.

Godman, D. (1991). *Be As You Are: The Teachings of Sri Ramana Maharshi.* Penguin.

Khalsa, GS & Bhajan, Y. (2008). *Breathwalk: Breathing Your Way to a Revitalised Body, Mind and Spirit.* Harmony.

Mooji (2012). *Before I Am: Second Edition.* Mooji Media.

Schucman, H. & Thetford, WN (1996). *A Course In Miracles: Combined Volume.* Viking.

Shannahoff-Khal, D. (2012). *Sacred Therapies: The Kundalini Meditation Handbook for Mental Health.* WW Norton & Company.

Spira, R. (2016). *The Transparency of Things.* Salisbury, UK: Non-Duality Press.

Yoga

Bhajan, Y. (2013). *The Chakras: Kundalini Yoga as Taught by Yogi Bhajan.* Kundalini Research Institute.

Bhajan, Y. & Kaur, HJ (2006). *Praana, Praanee, Praanayam.* Kundalini Research Institute.

Emerson, D. (2015). *Trauma-Sensitive Yoga in Therapy: Bringing the Body into Treatment.* WW Norton & Company.

Iyengar, BKS (2015). *Light on Yoga: The Definitive Guide to Yoga Practice.* Harper Thorsons.

Kaur, R. (2016). *The Body Temple: Kundalini Yoga for Body Acceptance, Eating Disorders & Radical Self-Love.* Spirit Voyage Records.

Kaur, S. (2016). *Original Light: The Morning Practice of Kundalini Yoga.* Sounds True.

Kaur Khalsa, SP (2001). *Kundalini Yoga: The Flow of Eternal*

Power—a Simple Guide to the Yoga of Awareness as Taught by Yogi Bhajan. GP Putnam's Sons.

Sivananda Yoga Vedanta Centre (2018). *Yoga: Your Home Practice Companion*. Dorling Kindersley.

Other Movement-Based Therapies

Feldenkrais, M. (1991). *Awareness Through Movement: Easy-To-Do Health Exercises to Improve Your Posture, Vision, Imagination, and Personal Awareness*. Thorsons.

Ogden, P., Minton, K. & Pain, C. (2006). *Trauma and the Body: A Sensorimotor Approach to Psychotherapy*. WW Norton & Company.

Van der Kolk, BA (2015). *The Body Keeps the Score: Brain, Mind, and Body in the Healing of Trauma*. Penguin.

Other

Damasio, A. (1999). *The Feeling of What Happens: Body and Emotion in the Making of Consciousness*. Harcourt.

Gerhardt, S. (2014). *Why Love Matters: How affection shapes a baby's brain*. Routledge.

Gilbert, P. (ed.) (2005). *Compassion: Conceptualisations, Research and Use in Psychotherapy*. Routledge.

Gilbert, P. (2010). *The Compassionate Mind: A New Approach to Life's Challenges*. New Harbinger Publications.

Siegel, D. (2016). *Mind: A Journey to the Heart of Being Human*. WW Norton & Company.

Also By This Author

Schnackenberg, N. (2016). *False Bodies, True Selves: Moving Beyond Appearance-Focused Identity Struggles and Returning to the True Self*. Karnac: Routledge.

Schnackenberg, N. & Petro, S. (2016). *Reflections on Body Dysmorphic Disorder: Stories of Courage, Determination and Hope*. Body Dysmorphic Disorder Foundation Publications.

Avenues of Support

Online Mindfulness Group for BDD and Associated Struggles: Run by meditation teacher, Richard Cox, and author, Nicole Schnackenberg. Monthly online meetings using Zoom. To be added to the mailing list, please email Richard Cox at richard@ timfreke.com.

The Body Dysmorphic Disorder Foundation (www. bddfoundation.org/): Offers support to individuals and their families in the form of face-to-face and Skype support groups. Their website is a rich source of information and contains personal stories of people diagnosed with BDD, as well as their family members.

OCD Action (www.ocdaction.org.uk/support-info/related-disorders/body-dysmorphia): Offers advice and support for people with obsessive-compulsive tendencies. They also provide information and advice about compulsive skin picking and hair pulling.

Beat (www.b-eat.co.uk/): Provides helplines, online support, and a network of self-help groups to assist young adults and people in the UK who are engaged in disordered eating practices. Helplines are for anyone who needs support and information.
Parents and Teachers Helpline: 0845 6341414
Helpline for Sufferers: 0845 6347650

The National Centre for Eating Disorders (https://eating-disorders.org.uk/): Offers treatment in person, over the phone, and via Skype. They also provide a database of specialist counsellors. The website contains a broad range of information on disordered eating and training materials/courses for professionals.

Men Get Eating Disorders Too (www.mengetedstoo.co.uk): A national charity offering peer support, advice, and workshops specifically for men.

Changing Faces (www.changingfaces.org.uk/): Offers self-help guides, support services, and workshops for people with visible differences.
Designated Support Helpline: 0300 012 0275

The Gender Trust (www.gendertrust.org.uk/): Provides support and an information centre for anyone with any questions or problems concerning their gender identity, or anyone whose loved one is struggling with gender identity issues. They offer help to people who might be transgender, transsexual, those who do not identify with the gender they were assigned at birth, or those who are simply unsure.

The Survivors Trust (www.thesurvivorstrust.org/): A national umbrella agency for over 135 specialist rape, sexual violence, and childhood sexual abuse support organisations throughout the UK and Ireland. They offer a comprehensive database of avenues of support for survivors and their families.

The Trauma Clinic (www.traumaclinic.org.uk/): Offers advice and treatment to people experiencing stress, anxiety, and depression in relation to past trauma.

For workshop information and to join the mailing list, visit www.nicoleschnackenberg.com.

About the Author

Nicole Schnackenberg is a psychologist, psychotherapist, a 200-hour Hatha yoga teacher, a Kundalini yoga teacher, a Director of the Yoga in Healthcare Alliance (YiHA), and a facilitator of the Eat Breathe Thrive yoga programme for food and body image issues.

Nicole currently divides her time between her clinical work in child and educational psychology, her position as a trustee of the Body Dysmorphic Disorder Foundation, and various forms of yoga teaching and yoga therapy. She has authored another book on the subject of appearance-focused identity struggles: *False Bodies, True Selves: Moving Beyond Appearance-Focused Identity Struggles and Returning to the True Self* (Karnac: Routledge) and co-edited a book on Body Dysmorphic Disorder: *Reflections on Body Dysmorphic Disorder: Stories of Courage, Determination and Hope* (the Body Dysmorphic Disorder Foundation).

BOOKS

SPIRITUALITY

O is a symbol of the world, of oneness and unity; this eye represents knowledge and insight. We publish titles on general spirituality and living a spiritual life. We aim to inform and help you on your own journey in this life.
If you have enjoyed this book, why not tell other readers by posting a review on your preferred book site?

Recent bestsellers from O-Books are:

Heart of Tantric Sex
Diana Richardson
Revealing Eastern secrets of deep love and intimacy to Western couples.
Paperback: 978-1-90381-637-0 ebook: 978-1-84694-637-0

Crystal Prescriptions
The A-Z guide to over 1,200 symptoms and their healing crystals
Judy Hall
The first in the popular series of six books, this handy little guide is packed as tight as a pill-bottle with crystal remedies for ailments.
Paperback: 978-1-90504-740-6 ebook: 978-1-84694-629-5

Take Me To Truth
Undoing the Ego
Nouk Sanchez, Tomas Vieira
The best-selling step-by-step book on shedding the Ego, using the teachings of A Course In Miracles.
Paperback: 978-1-84694-050-7 ebook: 978-1-84694-654-7

The 7 Myths about Love...Actually!
The journey from your HEAD to the HEART of your SOUL
Mike George
Smashes all the myths about LOVE.
Paperback: 978-1-84694-288-4 ebook: 978-1-84694-682-0

The Holy Spirit's Interpretation of the New Testament
A course in Understanding and Acceptance
Regina Dawn Akers
Following on from the strength of *A Course In Miracles*, NTI
teaches us how to experience the love and oneness of God.
Paperback: 978-1-84694-085-9 ebook: 978-1-78099-083-5

The Message of A Course In Miracles
A translation of the text in plain language
Elizabeth A. Cronkhite
A translation of *A Course in Miracles* into plain, everyday
language for anyone seeking inner peace. The companion
volume, *Practicing A Course In Miracles*, offers practical lessons
and mentoring.
Paperback: 978-1-84694-319-5 ebook: 978-1-84694-642-4

Thinker's Guide to God
Peter Vardy
An introduction to key issues in the philosophy of religion.
Paperback: 978-1-90381-622-6

Your Simple Path
Find happiness in every step
Ian Tucker
A guide to helping us reconnect with what is really important
in our lives.
Paperback: 978-1-78279-349-6 ebook: 978-1-78279-348-9

365 Days of Wisdom
Daily Messages To Inspire You Through The Year
Dadi Janki
Daily messages which cool the mind, warm the heart and guide
you along your journey.
Paperback: 978-1-84694-863-3 ebook: 978-1-84694-864-0

Body of Wisdom
Women's Spiritual Power and How it Serves
Hilary Hart
Bringing together the dreams and experiences of women across
the world with today's most visionary spiritual teachers.
Paperback: 978-1-78099-696-7 ebook: 978-1-78099-695-0

Dying to Be Free
From Enforced Secrecy to Near Death to True Transformation
Hannah Robinson
After an unexpected accident and near-death experience,
Hannah Robinson found herself radically transforming her life,
while a remarkable new insight altered her relationship with
her father, a practising Catholic priest.
Paperback: 978-1-78535-254-6 ebook: 978-1-78535-255-3

The Ecology of the Soul
A Manual of Peace, Power and Personal Growth for Real People
in the Real World
Aidan Walker
Balance your own inner Ecology of the Soul to regain your
natural state of peace, power and wellbeing.
Paperback: 978-1-78279-850-7 ebook: 978-1-78279-849-1

Not I, Not other than I
The Life and Teachings of Russel Williams
Steve Taylor, Russel Williams
The miraculous life and inspiring teachings of one of the
World's greatest living Sages.
Paperback: 978-1-78279-729-6 ebook: 978-1-78279-728-9

On the Other Side of Love
A Woman's Unconventional Journey Towards Wisdom
Muriel Maufroy
When life has lost all meaning, what do you do?
Paperback: 978-1-78535-281-2 ebook: 978-1-78535-282-9

Readers of ebooks can buy or view any of these bestsellers by clicking on the live link in the title. Most titles are published in paperback and as an ebook. Paperbacks are available in traditional bookshops. Both print and ebook formats are available online.

Find more titles and sign up to our readers' newsletter at http://www.johnhuntpublishing.com/mind-body-spirit

Follow us on Facebook at https://www.facebook.com/OBooks/ and Twitter at https://twitter.com/obooks